"*Globalism, Psychoanalysis, and the Integration of Eight Global Ideologies* is a provocative and ambitious contribution to contemporary debates about politics, ideology, and psychology. At a time when biological and rationalist explanations dominate the field, Robert Samuels makes a sustained case for the continued relevance of classical psychoanalysis—particularly Freudian metapsychology—in understanding political belief, polarization, and identification.

The book is both theoretically rigorous and clearly structured, offering a systematic framework that links eight distinct ideological positions to patterns of thought and relational dynamics rooted in depth psychology. Samuels engages directly with influential contemporary thinkers—from Zizek to Haidt—while situating his work in dialogue with historical figures such as Fromm and Aristotle. This integration of classical and contemporary perspectives makes the work particularly valuable for graduate students and scholars seeking a deeper, more nuanced understanding of ideology and its psychological underpinnings.

Written in a direct and accessible style, the book balances scholarly sophistication with readability, making complex ideas understandable without oversimplification. Whether one ultimately agrees with all of its claims or not, the work challenges prevailing assumptions and provides a timely, thought-provoking lens through which to examine the forces shaping political thought and social polarization today. It is a serious and significant contribution to psychoanalytic and political scholarship that invites reflection, discussion, and further research."

Karyne E. Messina, *psychoanalyst and a training analyst at the Washington Baltimore Center for Psychoanalysis, Washington, DC*

Globalism, Psychoanalysis, and the Integration of Eight Global Ideologies

Globalism, Psychoanalysis, and the Integration of Eight Global Ideologies argues that psychoanalysis helps us comprehend the different ideologies shaping our world today by examining eight distinct belief systems through their psychological and rhetorical roots, moving beyond simple Left–Right political polarization.

The work uses Freud's theory of psychology and politics to answer pressing contemporary questions including why people believe in conspiracy theories, why politics has become so polarized, and what drives people to join political cults. Each of the eight global ideologies is connected to specific childhood desires, relationships, and psychopathologies, offering a counter-narrative to evolutionary psychology approaches. The goal is to develop a new form of globalism that recognizes and integrates foundational human desires and different ideological frameworks rather than simply appealing to facts and reason alone.

This book will be a fascinating resource for psychoanalysts, as well as faculty and graduate students interested in psychoanalysis, political theory, and cultural rhetoric.

Robert Samuels holds doctorates in Psychoanalysis and English, and teaches advanced writing at the University of California, Santa Barbara. He is the author of twenty-five books, including *Trauma, Pedagogy, and the College Mental Health Crisis: Hysteria, Narcissism, and the Repression of Psychoanalysis* and *The Psychopathology of Political Ideologies*, both published by Routledge.

Globalism, Psychoanalysis, and the Integration of Eight Global Ideologies

Robert Samuels

Routledge
Taylor & Francis Group
LONDON AND NEW YORK

Designed cover image: Getty Images

First published 2027
by Routledge
4 Park Square, Milton Park, Abingdon, Oxon OX14 4RN

and by Routledge
605 Third Avenue, New York, NY 10158

Routledge is an imprint of the Taylor & Francis Group, an informa business

British Library Cataloguing in Publication Data
A catalogue record for this book is available from the British Library

ISBN: 9781041303237 (hbk)
ISBN: 9781041303213 (pbk)
ISBN: 9781003773948 (ebk)

DOI: 10.4324/9781003773948

Typeset in Times New Roman
by Taylor & Francis Books

Contents

Chapter 1

Introduction

According to Steven Pinker's *Enlightenment Now*, the driving forces behind global progress have been science, democracy, and humanism.[1] Due to the use of reason in the development of medicine and other technological advances, the global average lifespan has doubled in the last 150 years. Moreover, not only are people living longer, but they have more rights, protections, and freedom than ever before. However, the recent response to the COVID pandemic and the continued failure to fight climate change reveals that reason and correct knowledge are not enough: If people do not trust the information coming from scientists, governmental officials, and journalists, then they will not listen to the facts and do the right thing.

In order to help promote global progress, it is therefore necessary to understand what makes people trust science and what makes them mistrust experts. As we learn from the study of rhetoric, the use of logos or reason is not sufficient: People have to have trust (ethos), and they have to care (pathos) about the issue.[2] Moreover, they also need to feel that there will be a reward (catharsis) for their concern. It is thus necessary to understand these factors of persuasion (rhetoric) by gaining a better comprehension of reason, trust, concern, and reward. It is the argument of this book that psychoanalysis provides the most accurate and effective explanation of these key rhetorical social factors.

Psychoanalysis also helps us to comprehend the different ideologies shaping our world and blocking global progress.[3] Through the description of eight distinct ideologies, I hope to reveal the psychological roots of these belief systems. Instead of viewing the political world as a polarized conflict between the Left and the Right or liberal and conservative, I posit that we have to acknowledge the complex relationships among Right-wing, Leftist, conservative, liberal, traditional, center-Left, center-Right, and authoritarian ideologies. Furthermore, I relate each ideology to a specific psychopathology and fundamental human relationship.

In focusing on the psychopathological nature of political ideologies, my intent is not to make a moral judgment; instead, the goal is to show how specific ideologies attract individuals with particular unconscious defense

DOI: 10.4324/9781003773948-1

mechanisms, desires, and fears. The novelty of this approach is that it combines a close attention to political belief systems with a concern for individual subjectivity within a global context. Furthermore, I trace these psychological structures to early childhood mental processes and relationships.

As an aspect of the humanistic foundation of global progress, it is necessary to use psychoanalysis to critique the discourses that distort our understanding of ourselves and the social world around us. Psychoanalysis is key here because of its way of understanding human thought, emotions, motivation, and reason. Unlike the current push to use the theory of evolution to explain social institutions and individual thought, I turn to Freud's model of the human mind to reveal the unnatural and irrational foundations of consciousness and social order.[4]

The Freudian Theory of the Mind and Society

At the foundation of Freud's understanding of human thought and society is the notion that the main function of all societies is to regulate sex and aggression through the use of real and imagined violence, which he calls castration.[5] However, in order to make sure that people do not act on their impulses in a selfish, destructive way, it is necessary to impose social control when there is no authority present: In other words, people have to internalize morality and experience it as something coming from their own minds. Moreover, this form of internalization and control produces a paranoid mode of subjectivity since it is necessary for social subjects to constantly fear being punished by some invisible force.[6]

In his *Totem and Taboo,* Freud examined the work of anthropologists studying "primitive" societies, and he found that they often believe in animism, which is a belief in spirits.[7] He also found that these spirits represent the projection of an individual's conscience: In other words, the ghosts and spirits of dead people are seen as judging and punishing the living for their misdeeds.[8] Here, morality takes on a psychotic structure since thoughts are experienced as being the same as perceptions of the external world, and this process of projection is automatic and irrational since it is unintentional and makes a break with reality and reality-testing.[9] For instance, Freud found that paranoid psychotics think that they are constantly being observed because they perceive their internal conscience as coming from the outside.[10]

This theory of the social conscience is matched by Freud's theory of dreams. While Freud at first thought that all dreams represent a hallucinated fulfilment of an infantile sexual desire, he soon ran into the problem of what he called anxiety or punishment dreams.[11] What he discovered was that we often have nightmares that do not bring us pleasure or fulfilment: instead, we can be punished and criticized in our own dreams.[12] In fact, anxiety is often a response to the fear of potential harm caused by negative judgments.

Moreover, dreams show us how we do not completely control our own minds, and the representations in our dreams are scenes that rely on symbolic associations, substitutions, and displacement.[13] Thus, on the level of the primary process of our minds, our thoughts are unintentional, irrational, and indirect. In fact, the use of indirect representation points to a form of automatic poetry that employs rhetorical figures, like metaphor.[14]

It turns out that if we want to truly understand human thought, social order, and ideology, we have to acknowledge the psychotic foundation of both the mind and society. Although this sounds like an absurd argument, we should remember that right before Descartes states his famous "I think therefore, I am," he posits that we never know if we are awake or dreaming, but what we do know is that in both states, we are thinking.[15] Thus, if we define human consciousness by thought, we must conclude that consciousness is fundamentally unintentional, irrational, and indirect, and it is this conception of consciousness that is repressed by most neuroscientists, evolutionary psychologists, and philosophers.[16]

Although Freud calls the initial stage of social organization animistic and primitive, I prefer to use the term traditional to avoid stigmatization and to clarify the relationship between morality and social rituals. From this perspective, a traditional ideology is one that is unintentional, irrational, and indirect and which relies on the processes of projection and introjection.[17] While projection explains how internal thoughts are transformed into the perception of external objects, introjection deals with how external content is experienced as coming from the inner self.[18] Furthermore, what explains the difference between actual psychosis and "normal" thought is the level of certainty: In psychosis, there is no room for doubt or questioning of the reality of one's consciousness since one's thoughts are experienced as perceptions of immediate reality.[19] On the other hand, what makes reason possible is the ability to test the reality of our own thoughts.[20] I claim that if we do not grasp this psychoanalytic understanding of human consciousness and social organization, then we cannot understand ourselves or the political ideologies around us.

Not only does Freud's theory of the paranoid super-ego help us to comprehend what makes people submit to social norms and rules when no authority is directly present, but his theory of the primary processes also explains his conception of infantile subjectivity. According to the founder of psychoanalysis, the first way that a person tries to satisfy their own desires is by imagining the repetition of a past scene of satisfaction. Thus, through a process of hallucinating a symbolic scene, one is able to satisfy unmet wishes, and this form of imagination causes a radical break with reality. Furthermore, we can consider human imagination as our greatest strength and our greatest weakness. Since we can imagine things that do not exist, we can create new knowledge and new ways of solving problems, yet this break from reality also makes us prone to destructive delusions and manipulation from others.

The fact that our minds can transcend material reality plays a key role in the internalization of social control: Due to the fact that we can imagine things that are not directly present, we can imagine social punishments and rewards when we are all alone. Thus, the fundamental desire for satisfactions opens us up to social control. From this perspective, traditional ideology takes advantage of our desire for satisfaction as we automatically imagine the fulfilment of our wishes.

Competing Ideologies

The traditional way of thinking is sometimes coupled with the need for salvation, which in its extreme form can lead to the ideology of authoritarianism. While every society needs some level of authority, the unregulated form of this human value results in the total submission of the individual to a particular person or ideal. For Freud, what we find in transference is the transferring of power from the individual to the Other, and this type of relationship is based on a desire to escape freedom, responsibility, guilt, and shame.[21] After all, if the Other is in control, then the individual cannot be blamed.

While the ideology of authoritarianism requires a loss of individual freedom, libertarian ideology is centered on the fantasy of the total liberty and enjoyment of the isolated individual.[22] Thus, by celebrating free markets and free speech, Right-wing ideology concentrates on the freedom of the individual to act on his own desires and drives without restraint. Ironically, in contemporary global politics, the opposing forces of liberty and authority are often united in a coalition, which tends to use a shared fear and hatred of the Left and liberalism to bring together these opposing values: In other words, authoritarians and libertarians bond together through a shared opposition.

Since humans are driven to be free and independent, we cannot simply reject this desire, yet we need to learn how to balance each value in an integrated system. For example, the key conflict in modernity is between individual freedom and collective equality.[23] Due to the fact that equal treatment requires submitting oneself to a universal law, the freedom of the individual is limited within liberal democratic ideology. Yet, we cannot simply remove freedom from our social structures because people are motivated by drives that promote free will and the pursuit of happiness. In fact, modern capitalism can be seen as focused on an ideology of individual liberty—even though it relies on social exchange, a shared currency, and legal guarantees.[24]

Since modern equality and freedom do not remove all human suffering, it is necessary to have progressive social movements based on recognizing the suffering of the disadvantaged. From this perspective, Left-wing ideologies tend to focus on accommodating oppressed minority groups.[25] As we shall see, in its extreme form, this call for special help can result in a victim complex where the innocent self is opposed by an evil Other.[26] In this ideological structure, the self escapes any criticism, and all vengeance is justified.

For the person who identifies as being a victim, there is a strong desire to have suffering recognized in a hysterical psychopathology, but in the case of narcissism and center-Left politics, the desire is to have a special self admired by others in order to overcome feelings of shame and insecurity.[27] In what is often mistaken as a form of liberalism, Left-leaning centrists want to signal their virtue in order to hide anti-social drives from others and their own self.

For people on the center-Right, we often find an unconscious rationalization of privilege and a naturalizing of the social order. While they desire to be recognized as being neutral, liberal, and democratic, they actually take advantage of social inequality.[28] In this ideology, we often see an investment in evolutionary psychology, neuroscience, and a belief in the natural foundations of social inequality and hierarchy. Furthermore, people on the center-Right like to show how they believe in science, reason, open debate, and free speech, yet they often seek to cash in on their fake liberalism as they pursue, individual, anti-social drives.[29]

These false "liberals" desire to engage in the rewards of capitalism and self-promotion, but they also want to maintain a reputation of being fair and innocent. Thus, one of the things that distinguishes the center-Right from liberalism is that a key principle of modern liberal democracy and science is the need to base one's judgments on a neutral analysis of empirical evidence.[30] Therefore, equality is the central value of liberalism because science and democratic law require taking a universal perspective void of bias. In contrast, for the person performing center-Right politics, the main value is to protect an innocent image of the self while one represses the benefits one gets from social privilege.

Since humans also value self-protection, there is a conservative ideology and politics centered on the call to identify and eliminate potential risks.[31] Often, this phobic pathology relies on finding scapegoats as substitute causes for social ills.[32] As a way of protecting oneself and others against real and imagined threats, conservativism does not call for an idealized savior; rather, the desire for protection results in a call for law and order coupled with strong borders and discriminatory practices in order to prevent change or an encounter with the unknown or foreign.

A central claim of this book is that we cannot simply wish way the fundamental desires shaping these distinct ideologies, and so we need to find a way to moderate and balance these essential human values. Moreover, if we want to pursue global progress through the use of science, reason, and democracy, we have to realize that people will not be persuaded by appeals to facts and truth alone; instead, it is necessary to develop a mode of globalism that recognizes and integrates the foundational human desires with the different ideologies and rhetorical strategies shaping globalism today.

Book Outline

One of the strong claims of this book is that if we do not recognize the need to understand and integrate these different human values, then we will be unable to build a truly just and effective system of global politics. Since, as I document in Chapter 2, we have global problems that need global solutions, we must develop a new form of consciousness around a global mode of solidarity and understanding. However, while Steven Pinker argues that the key to this change is to affirm the importance of modern democratic equality and scientific reason, I show how this liberal ideology is not enough.[33]

To help examine the different ideologies and relational desires shaping our world today, I turn in Chapter 3 to Jonathan Haidt's *The Righteousness Mind* where he ties five different ideologies to specific moral taste buds.[34] Although I reject his effort to naturalize political belief systems, I do see his work as a starting point to differentiate diverse ideologies. By adding a Freudian perspective, the goal is to connect each ideology to a different social relation and psychopathology.

In Chapter 4, we turn to the *Ideological Brain* by Leor Zmigrod.[35] Here we find another attempt to tie ideology to mental processes, but the problem with this work is that it uses a simplistic binary logic to equate the mind with the brain as it reproduces a polarized discourse. In focusing on the difference between rigid and flexible mental functioning, she is able to apply a narcissistic form of virtue signaling as she clearly identifies with the ideal of flexibility against the debased notion of rigidity. What is most revealing about her discourse is that she displays unintentionally the connection between the narcissistic desire for admiration and the center-Left politics of virtue signaling.

Chapter 5 discusses the roots of center-Right ideology by analyzing Aristotle's *Rhetoric*. [36] This work is so important because it reveals how obsessionals seek to naturalize and rationalize social hierarchies by basing them on a supposed natural order, which is really a reflection of the subject's own privilege and idealized character traits. Thus, when Aristotle argues that it is natural for men to dominate women and for thought to be favored over emotion, he is simply idealizing his own sense of being a masculine intellectual.

Chapter 6 places the eight main ideologies within a historical context by analyzing Erich Fromm's *Escape from Freedom*. [37] One of the benefits of this work is that he combines psychoanalysis with sociology and history as he tries to answer the question of why so many people submit to authoritarian rule. Fromm also examine how modernity acts to generate anxiety as older forms of protection are replaced by a capitalist system of isolated individuals.

In Chapter 7, I focus on Freud's *Totem and Taboo* and *Group Psychology and the Analysis of the Ego* in order to provide a psychoanalytic framework for traditional ideology. This work also helps us to understand why people believe in conspiracy theories and different forms of spirituality. One of the main goals here is to demonstrate the way projection, introjection, and polarization are used to structure the content of most belief systems.

Chapter 8 continues this examination of Freud's contribution to our understanding of ideology through a critical interpretation of *Moses and Monotheism* and *The Ego and the Id.* [38] The goal here is to connect each ideology and social relation to a particular mental agency. This effort to recognize all of the different values and mental processes shaping human thought and social beliefs pushes us to call for a balanced and integrated model of globalism both as a form of politics and a mode of consciousness. Finally, the conclusion of the book returns to the main themes in order to outline what the philosophy, psychology, and politics of globalism should look like.

Notes

1 Pinker, Steven. *Enlightenment now: The case for reason, science, humanism, and progress.* Penguin, 2018.
2 Samuels, Robert. *Žižek and the rhetorical unconscious: Global politics, philosophy, and subjectivity.* Springer Nature, 2020.
3 Samuels, Robert. *The psychopathology of political ideologies.* Routledge, 2021.
4 Samuels, Robert. *Psychoanalyzing the politics of the new brain sciences.* Springer, 2017.
5 Freud, Sigmund. *Civilization and its discontents.* Broadview Press, 2015.
6 Traetta, Luigi, and Federica Doronzo. "Super-ego after Freud: A lesson not to Be forgotten." *Elementa: Intersections between Philosophy, Epistemology and Empirical Perspectives* 1.1–2 (2022): 153–161.
7 Moser, Franz. "Beyond Sigmund Freud's Totem and Taboo vision for the future-the omnipotence of thought." *International Journal of Foresight and Innovation Policy* 13.3–4 (2018): 187–194.
8 Hurry, Anne, Jack Novick, and Kerry Kelly Novick. "Freud's concept of projection." *Journal of Child Psychotherapy* 4.2 (1976): 75–88.
9 Zuk, Gerald H., and Carmen V. Zuk. "When more is better than less: Three theories of psychosis—projection, double bind, and possession." *Contemporary Family Therapy* 20.1 (1998): 3–13.
10 Freud, Sigmund. "Some neurotic mechanisms in jealousy, paranoia, and homosexuality." In Nancy Burke (ed.), *Gender and envy.* Routledge, 2014: 213–220.
11 Freud, Sigmund. *On dreams.* Good Press, 2025.
12 Fisher, Charles, et al. "A psychophysiological study of nightmares." *Journal of the American Psychoanalytic Association* 18.4 (1970): 747–782.
13 Robbins, Michael. "Another look at dreaming: Disentangling Freud's primary and secondary process theories." *Journal of the American Psychoanalytic Association* 52.2 (2004): 355–384.
14 Edelson, Jonathan T. "Freud's use of metaphor." *The Psychoanalytic Study of the Child* 38.1 (1983): 17–59.
15 Descartes, René. "Descartes's discourse on method." *Ratio et Fides: A Preliminary Introduction to Philosophy for Theology* 109 (2018).
16 Samuels, Robert. *The psychoanalytic understanding of consciousness, free will, language, and reason: What makes us human?* Routledge, 2023.

17 Bowdler, Sandra. "Freud and archaeology." *Anthropological Forum* 7.3 (1996).
18 Knight, Robert P. "Introjection, projection and identification." *The Psychoanalytic Quarterly* 9.3 (1940): 334–341.
19 Kovar, Leo. "A reconsideration of paranoia." *Psychiatry* 29.3 (1966): 289–305.
20 Freud, Sigmund. "Formulations on the two principles of mental functioning." In James Strachey (ed.), *The standard edition of the complete psychological works of Sigmund Freud.* Vol. 12. Hogarth Press, 1953–1974: 213–226.
21 Freud, Sigmund. *Group psychology and the analysis of the ego.* Hogarth Press, 1949.
22 Samuels, Warren J. "The myths of liberty and the realities of the corporate state: A review article." *Journal of Economic Issues* 10.4 (1976): 923–942.
23 Heller, Agnes. "Rights, modernity, democracy." In Drucilla Cornell, Michel Rosenfeld, and David Gray Carlson (eds.), *Deconstruction and the possibility of justice.* Routledge, 2016: 346–360.
24 Youngmevittaya, Wanpat. "Ethics, freedom, and capitalism: A critical account of Marxism and libertarianism." *Journal of Social Sciences Naresuan University* 12.2 (2016): 71–111.
25 Samuels, Robert. "Pathos, hysteria, and the Left." In Robert Samuels, *Žižek and the rhetorical unconscious: Global politics, philosophy, and subjectivity.* Springer, 2020: 33–47.
26 Jacoby, Tami Amanda. "A theory of victimhood: Politics, conflict and the construction of victim-based identity." *Millennium* 43.2 (2015): 511–530.
27 Samuels, Robert. "(Liberal) narcissism." In Yannis Stavrakakis (ed.), *Routledge handbook of psychoanalytic political theory.* Routledge, 2019: 151–161.
28 Gidron, Noam, and Daniel Ziblatt. "Center-Right political parties in advanced democracies." *Annual Review of Political Science* 22.1 (2019): 17–35.
29 Jost, John T., et al. "Ideology and the limits of self-interest: System justification motivation and conservative advantages in mass politics." *Translational Issues in Psychological Science* 3.3 (2017): e1.
30 Fukuyama, Francis. "Liberal democracy as a global phenomenon." *Political Science & Politics* 24.4 (1991): 659–664.
31 Helminen, Vilja, Marko Elovainio, and Markus Jokela. "Clinical symptoms of anxiety disorders as predictors of political attitudes: A prospective cohort study." *International Journal of Psychology* 57.2 (2022): 181–189.
32 Gentry, Caron E. "Anxiety and the creation of the scapegoated other." *Critical Studies on Security* 3.2 (2015): 133–146.
33 Pinker, Steven. *Enlightenment now: The case for reason, science, humanism, and progress.* Penguin, 2018.
34 Haidt, Jonathan. *The righteous mind: Why good people are divided by politics and religion.* Vintage, 2012.
35 Zmigrod, Leor. *The ideological brain.* Henry Holt, 2025.
36 Cope, Edward Meredith, and John Edwin Sandys, eds. *Aristotle: rhetoric.* Vol. 2. Cambridge University Press, 2010.
37 Fromm, Erich. *Escape from freedom.* Henry Holt, 1969.
38 Freud, Sigmund. *Moses and monotheism.* Sanzani Edizioni, 2023.

Chapter 2

Reason and Equality

Steven Pinker's False Path to Globalism

After reading Steven Pinker's *Enlightenment Now*, I became convinced that the key to developing a truly global society is to follow the universal principles of science and democracy.[1] After all, we can think of globalization as the process of spreading the same modern liberal democratic and scientific ideology to the entire planet.[2] However, this push to make the world more reasonable runs into a problem: Humans tend to have specific desires that are not satisfied by the push for equality and truth. The question then is do we try to simply replace these non-rational and non-universal values, or do we have to find a way to integrate and balance these different factors?

Liberalism and Its Discontents

Since most humans want to be free to make their own choices and pursue their own pleasure, we can say that it would make no sense to insist on a single system of strict authority where everyone was motivated to simply submit to a higher authority or some universal system.[3] Furthermore, as Pinker himself notes, any attempt to make society more fair or rational runs into the problem of dealing with other basic human desires: "The ideals of the Enlightenment are products of human reason, but they always struggle with other strands of human nature: loyalty to tribe, deference to authority, magical thinking, the blaming of misfortune on evildoers" (*EN*: 5). As Pinker highlights, the great promoters of modern reason and equality thought that the new ideals of the Enlightenment could simply replace older ideals and values, yet history has shown that this replacement has been impossible to achieve.[4]

One of the main reasons why we have been unable to build a global society based on universal human rights and scientific reason is that other competing ideologies are shaped by core human desires related to specific types of childhood relationships. Thus, as Freud insists, when a baby cries because it is feeling discomfort, it wants someone to make it feel better.[5] In other words, suffering calls for accommodation. Moreover, once a caregiver helps make the suffering go away, the person who helped the subject is idealized in

DOI: 10.4324/9781003773948-2

a relationship based on the desire for salvation. As a mode of transference, the person who desires help transfers responsibility and agency over to the helper, and this basic human relationship becomes the source of authority and idealization, which in its extreme form shapes authoritarian ideology.[6]

Although we may wish to move beyond any type of relationship or politics based on idealized authority, it would be wrong to ignore the fundamental relational desire for being helped by another person. What we need to do is to integrate this call to transfer responsibility to others with different human desires, like the call for autonomy and freedom.[7] Even though we often find political coalitions built on the combination of individual liberty (Right-wing libertarianism) and submissive authoritarianism, it is vital to recognize that freedom and authority are inherently opposed. In fact, this opposition is often overcome in political parties by uniting around a shared hated object.[8] For instance, by demonizing immigrants or Leftists, opposite political ideologies are able to bond together.[9] This use of a phobic objects by conservatives who desire protection is itself enabled by the activation of traditional conspiracy theories and magical thinking.[10] Thus, the reason why people are not afraid of what really threatens them and society is that their minds are able to substitute a real threat with an imagined one.[11]

This use of imagination in ideology points to the essential conflict between the desire for symbolic order and the call for equality. While conspiracy theories can help people to imagine that they know what is happening through the use of magical thinking, with modern science and democracy we rely on the separation of fact from fiction and the imposition of universal ideals.[12] In fact, for Pinker, what in part defines the modern Enlightenment is its opposition to traditional modes of belief:

> To the Enlightenment thinkers the escape from ignorance and superstition showed how mistaken our conventional wisdom could be, and how the methods of science—skepticism, fallibilism, open debate, and empirical testing—are a paradigm of how to achieve reliable knowledge. (*EN*: 10)

Similar to Freud's argument that individuals have to learn how to replace the primary processes with the reality principle, Pinker insists that at the heart of modern science, we find a rejection of superstition and other modes of magical thinking.[13]

Coupled with the promotion of science and democratic law, Pinker bases the ideology of modern liberalism on the philosophy of humanism:

> The idea of a universal human nature brings us to a third theme, humanism. The thinkers of the Age of Reason and the Enlightenment saw an urgent need for a secular foundation for morality, because they were haunted by a historical memory of centuries of religious carnage:

> the Crusades, the Inquisition, witch hunts, the European wars of religion.
>
> (*EN*: 10)

From this perspective, the path to a system of universal human rights and scientific reason leads to the elimination of religion as an authoritarian ideology.[14] However, history tells another story since even Enlightenment thinkers like Descartes still showed a commitment to religion even while they attempted to limit the call to submit to unquestioned authorities.[15]

Although some argue that the problem is that the modern Enlightenment did not go far enough because it was afraid of the consequences of attacking Christianity directly, a psychoanalytic explanation argues that the main reason why science was not able to replace faith was that people have a desire for salvation and meaning.[16] In other words, the hunger for truth has to be balanced against the call for trust since in order to take science seriously, one has to first trust the experts and then try to verify the results.[17] Moreover, as Pinker describes in his discussion of humanism, the quest for a society based on universal evidence and equality has to contend with other basic relational desires:

> They laid that foundation in what we now call humanism, which privileges the well-being of individual men, women, and children over the glory of the tribe, race, nation, or religion. It is individuals, not groups, who are sentient—who feel pleasure and pain, fulfillment and anguish. Whether it is framed as the goal of providing the greatest happiness for the greatest number or as a categorical imperative to treat people as ends rather than means, it was the universal capacity of a person to suffer and flourish, they said, that called on our moral concern.
>
> (*EN*: 11)

This passage reflects an inherent conflict in our understanding of modern liberalism, which is the tension between universality and individuality. While modern liberal democracy is centered on equal treatment under the law, libertarian ideology promotes the individual over society.[18] This opposition can also be found in the fundamental divide between modern capitalism and modern democracy as one ideology caters to the desire for individual liberty, while the other one is focused on applying the law and science in an impersonal, disinterested way.[19]

Balancing Ideological Desires

Since we cannot simply eliminate the desire for fairness or the call for freedom, we have to find a way to balance and moderate each demand. Furthermore, as the passage above indicates, not only do people want to discover the truth of the world, but they also want to find meaning and a higher purpose as they seek recognition for their own goodness and suffering. Interestingly, Pinker posits that at the heart of the humanistic desire for universal justice and scientific truth, we find sympathy as a fundamental aspect of human nature:

> Fortunately, human nature prepares us to answer that call. That is because we are endowed with the sentiment of sympathy, which they also called benevolence, pity, and commiseration. Given that we are equipped with the capacity to sympathize with others, nothing can prevent the circle of sympathy from expanding from the family and tribe to embrace all of humankind, particularly as reason goads us into realizing that there can be nothing uniquely deserving about ourselves or any of the groups to which we belong. We are forced into cosmopolitanism: accepting our citizenship in the world.
>
> (*EN*: 11)

From this perspective, the path to globalism passes through sympathy as a basic aspect of human nature; however, it is unclear if a universal human nature actually exists, and the push for universal human rights is not necessarily based on sympathy. In fact, I would argue that the imposition of an impersonal, impartial legal system is an artificial social construct that seeks to remove feelings like sympathy from the unbiased judgment of the facts.[20] Moreover, as we see in the ideological battle between the liberal emphasis on equality and the Left-wing focus on empathy and special accommodation, sympathy is not the same as universality.[21]

From the view of liberal democracy, the desire for truth and fairness is answered by the formation of social institutions determined by reason.[22] However, Pinker does not fully endorse this need to actualize democratic and scientific ideals in shared social organizations:

> The ideal of progress also should not be confused with the 20th-century movement to re-engineer society for the convenience of technocrats and planners, which the political scientist James Scott calls Authoritarian High Modernism. The movement denied the existence of human nature, with its messy needs for beauty, nature, tradition, and social intimacy. Starting from a "clean tablecloth," the modernists designed urban renewal projects that replaced vibrant neighborhoods with freeways, high-rises, windswept plazas, and brutalist architecture. "Mankind will be reborn," they theorized, and "live in an ordered relation to the whole." Though these developments were sometimes linked to the word progress, the usage was ironic: "progress" unguided by humanism is not progress.
>
> (*EN*: 11–12)

In this rejection of technocrats and planners, Pinker reveals why it is hard to base a society on pure reason or universal rules: Since people desire tradition, beauty, and social intimacy, they resist the imposition of what they see as an impersonal law or social order. In other words, people have several different relational desires that cannot be replaced by a society based on reason and equality alone.

For Pinker, the term "human nature" is employed in order to point to some type of biological determinism, and yet, Freud shows how humans are always shaped by a mixture of psychology, biology, culture, and the unconscious.[23] In fact, the belief in a natural order forms the essence of the center-Right ideology and the desire for a fixed social system predetermined by nature.[24]Interestingly, even though Pinker at times does seem to believe in the combination of universal equality and a naturalized hierarchy, he also recognizes the need for modern institutions that are socially constructed:

> Rather than trying to shape human nature, the Enlightenment hope for progress was concentrated on human institutions. Human-made systems like governments, laws, schools, markets, and international bodies are a natural target for the application of reason to human betterment.
>
> (*EN*: 12)

Since social institutions go beyond nature and evolution, they are built out of necessary but impossible ideals—like equality and neutrality.[25]

From the perspective of modern liberal ideology, the government should not be based on religion, race, or nationalism; instead, universal human rights and empirical science rely on an implicit social contract:

> In this way of thinking, government is not a divine fiat to reign, a synonym for "society," or an avatar of the national, religious, or racial soul. It is a human invention, tacitly agreed to in a social contract, designed to enhance the welfare of citizens by coordinating their behavior and discouraging selfish acts that may be tempting to every individual but leave everyone worse off. As the most famous product of the Enlightenment, the Declaration of Independence, put it, in order to secure the right to life, liberty, and the pursuit of happiness, governments are instituted among people, deriving their just powers from the consent of the governed.
>
> (*EN*: 11)

What is interested in this reference to the Declaration of Independence is that it points to an inherent conflict between the need for shared rules and the individual's pursuit of pleasure and liberty, which are the foundations of a libertarian ideology.[26] There is thus a central tension in liberal democracy and modernity itself since we find two opposing relational desires and ideologies: On the one hand we have the desire for fairness and the giving up of selfish impulses, and on the other hand, we have the libertarian pursuit of individual freedom and pleasure. The battle between the pleasure principle and the reality principle is then foundational to the modern world.[27]

Reason and Global Progress

As Pinker insists, the Enlightenment has been the driving force behind global progress and the amazing increase in human lifespans since 1850, yet this combination of scientific reason and democratic law is in a constant battle with other human relational desires:

> If there's anything the Enlightenment thinkers had in common, it was an insistence that we energetically apply the standard of reason to understanding our world, and not fall back on generators of delusion like faith, dogma, revelation, authority, charisma, mysticism, divination, visions, gut feelings, or the hermeneutic parsing of sacred texts.
>
> (*EN*: 8)

Even though the world has become more secular over the last two centuries, religion still plays a powerful role in many people's lives, and so the modern push for reason as the way to understand the world has only been partially successful.[28] What Pinker does not fully address is why it is so difficult to replace faith, dogma, authority, and mysticism with abstract reason and universal rights.

I argue that if we want to have a more just and fair global order, then we have to learn how to moderate and balance the different relational desires and ideologies shaping human psychology. In other terms, we cannot simply hope that reason will eventually replace older ideologies since these belief systems are determined by basic human desires developed out of crucial childhood experiences. Just as Freud tried to match the development of civilization with the development of the individual, we need to understand how psychology and culture relate to each other.[29]As we shall see in the following passage, Pinker, at times, does realize this necessity to combine philosophy, psychology, and sociology:

> Thinkers such as Kant, Baruch Spinoza, Thomas Hobbes, David Hume, and Adam Smith were inquisitive psychologists and all too aware of our irrational passions and foibles. They insisted that it was only by calling out the common sources of folly that we could hope to overcome them. The deliberate application of reason was necessary precisely because our common habits of thought are not particularly reasonable.
>
> (*EN*: 11)

Similar to Freud's model of critical introspection, these modern philosophers realized that the only way to promote reason was to explore the reason of unreason. However, what is missing from most philosophy is the Freudian insight that we are not fully in control of our own thoughts and desires.[30] As we discover through the analysis of dreams and slips of the tongue, people often say more than they want to say and also think things they do not intend. Furthermore, the discovery of unreason by reason is undermined by the human tendency for self-deception.[31] As the foundation of the unconscious, repression entails the idea that humans hide from themselves their own feelings and thoughts if these mental representations harm an idealized self-image.[32] In fact, I have defined center-Left ideology as a form of narcissism because the focus is on gaining admiration for one's good intentions in order to repress feelings of shame, guilt, and hostility.[33]

Like many other academic philosophers and psychologists, Pinker himself may be attempting to signal his virtue by prioritizing reason and fairness above other human desires. Therefore, while it may be true that a world based on reason would be more fair and accurate, the push to eliminate all of the other relational desires results in a repression of the very things that make us human.[34] Ironically, at the very moment Pinker idealizes reason as the cause for global progress, he falls back on a traditional version of natural order: "Evolution left us with another burden: our cognitive, emotional, and moral faculties are adapted to individual survival and reproduction in an archaic environment, not to universal thriving in a modern one" (*EN*: 25). Even though the theory of evolution is clearly a modern scientific discovery, it is often used as a way of returning to a naturalized traditional order.[35] Thus, by saying that evolution makes us focus on individual survival and not life in the modern world, Pinker replaces relational desires with inherited mental programs.

Projection, Introjection, and the Primary Processes

Through his compulsive return to explanations based on some imagined natural order, Pinker undermines his own desire to base society on reason:

> People are by nature illiterate and innumerate, quantifying the world by "one, two, many" and by rough guesstimates. They understand physical things as having hidden essences that obey the laws of sympathetic magic or voodoo rather than physics and biology: objects can reach across time and space to affect things that resemble them or that had been in contact with them in the past (remember the beliefs of pre–Scientific Revolution Englishmen). They think that words and thoughts can impinge on the physical world in prayers and curses. They underestimate the prevalence of coincidence. They generalize from paltry samples, namely their own experience, and they reason by stereotype, projecting the typical traits of a group onto any individual that belongs to it. They infer causation from correlation. They think holistically, in black and white, and physically,

> treating abstract networks as concrete stuff. They are not so much intuitive scientists as intuitive lawyers and politicians, marshaling evidence that confirms their convictions while dismissing evidence that contradicts them. They overestimate their own knowledge, understanding, rectitude, competence, and luck.
>
> (*EN*: 26)

What Pinker is describing here is precisely the type of thinking that dominates in what Freud calls the primary processes and "primitive" animistic cultures.[36] Through the use of symbolic association, substitutions, and displacements, we seek out order in a chaotic world, and by projecting our thoughts onto external reality, we confuse our internal mental representations with the natural world.[37] Moreover, this process of projection is combined with introjection, which entails the way we treat the ideas of others as if they were our own ideas.[38] In fact, Freud argues that the formation of a conscience (super-ego) is determined by the internalization of social morality, and this morality itself reinforces social hierarchies.[39]

Although it would represent progress for us to replace our primary processes with abstract reason and reality testing, this is an unrealistic goal since part of our minds function through the use of magical thinking and symbolism.[40] Furthermore, our social orders are based on the use of symbolic representations to regulate sex and violence in the goal of promoting stability and safety.[41] As Freud argues in *Totem and Taboo*, the primary form of civilization is founded on the use of irrational, indirect, and unintentional thoughts, and this type of traditional ideology cannot be simply wished away or fully repressed.[42] It is also vital to realize that the desire for order and meaning is often coupled with a call for protection and security: "People demonize those they disagree with, attributing differences of opinion to stupidity and dishonesty. For every misfortune they seek a scapegoat. They see morality as a source of grounds for condemning rivals and mobilizing indignation against them" (*EN*: 26). While traditional societies have a strict moral order that clearly distinguishes between good and evil, us and them, and the powerful and the disempowered, they also tend to designate scapegoats in order to displace fear onto collective targets.[43] In this phobic, conservative ideology, the desire for protection is coupled with an irrational sense of risk and threat.[44] Traditional and conservative ideologies thus often come together because they unite the desire for order with the fear of disorder: As we find in many modes of prejudice, the outsider becomes the symbol for what prevents the social order from being complete and ideal.

While Pinker does realize that knowledge can be both delusional and truthful, he tends to fall back onto a modern idealization of thought:

> Thanks to language, ideas are not just abstracted and combined inside the head of a single thinker but can be pooled across a community of

> thinkers. Thomas Jefferson explained the power of language with the help of an analogy: "He who receives an idea from me, receives instruction himself without lessening mine; as he who lights his taper at mine, receives light without darkening me."
>
> (*EN*: 27)

The problem with this Enlightenment idealization of thought is that it can function to repress the ways thoughts are often irrational, unintentional, and indirect.[45] Therefore, even when thoughts are shared through language on a social basis that does not mean that the knowledge is accurate or based on reality testing. In fact, one of the fundamental desires humans have is to be able to predict and understand the world in order to avoid threats and risks, and this call for protection leads to a conservative phobic ideology.

Liberal Ideology and Its Other

As Pinker insists, our thoughts can do great harm, but they can also lead to great good:

> So for all the flaws in human nature, it contains the seeds of its own improvement, as long as it comes up with norms and institutions that channel parochial interests into universal benefits. Among those norms are free speech, nonviolence, cooperation, cosmopolitanism, human rights, and an acknowledgment of human fallibility, and among the institutions are science, education, media, democratic government, international organizations, and markets. Not coincidentally, these were the major brainchildren of the Enlightenment.
>
> (*EN*: 28)

In this description of the ideology of the modern liberal Enlightenment, Pinker emphasizes the desire for universality in both the law and in science.[46] He also posits that the same relational desire should structure social institutions like journalism, education, and even economic markets. However, what undermines this ideology of liberal universality is that modern capitalism is focused on the desire for individual liberation and satisfaction and not the need for universal equality.[47]

In Pinker's strong defense of liberal ideology, he seeks to counter the notion that the supposed universality of this discourse hides the promotion of a particular demographic group and culture:

> Indeed, a common criticism of the Enlightenment project—that it is a Western invention, unsuited to the world in all its diversity—is doubly wrongheaded. For one thing, all ideas have to come from somewhere, and their birthplace has no bearing on their merit. Though many

> Enlightenment ideas were articulated in their clearest and most influential form in 18th-century Europe and America, they are rooted in reason and human nature, so any reasoning human can engage with them.
>
> (*EN*: 29)

Once again, this emphasis on human nature seeks to replace relational desires with a type of natural order; however, as Freud makes clear, social organizations are structured by an interaction between culture, biology, psychology, and the unconscious, and so it is misleading to point to some type of instinctual sociality in order to account for the formation of vital global social institutions.[48]

Nationalism, Tradition, and Authority

Like many other Enlightenment philosophers, Pinker reveals how religion can undermine modern liberal ideology:

> Religions also commonly clash with humanism whenever they elevate some moral good above the well-being of humans, such as accepting a divine savior, ratifying a sacred narrative, enforcing rituals and taboos, proselytizing other people to do the same, and punishing or demonizing those who don't.
>
> (*EN*: 30)

I believe that this description demonstrates how center-Right philosophers and psychologists often repress the differences among traditional, conservative, and authoritarian ideologies. While it is true that many religions rely on tradition and purification rituals, what distinguishes the monotheistic belief systems is the idealization of a single higher power coupled with the suspension of critical thinking.[49] Moreover, the promotion of a moral good is derived from the traditional need to create a social order by strictly determining what is good and evil. In turn, conservative ideology is triggered when a particular out-group becomes demonized so that the in-group can protect itself against an imagined risk or threat. Thus, even though many religions combine together conservative, traditional, and authoritarian ideologies together, it is important to see how each one of these ideologies is based on a specific relational desire that has been taken to the extreme.[50]

For the most part, politics involves bringing together different ideologies in order to enhance power and support, and so what we often find is that extreme versions of different relational desires are linked together under the banner of one party or movement.[51] The solution to this problem is to understand that people have different relational desires that need to be recognized, yet it is also important to moderate and balance these desires.

For instance, in the following passage, Pinker attempts to describe the distinction between modern liberal reason and nationalism, but his analysis is undermined by his failure to clearly separate conservative, authoritarian, and traditional ideologies:

> A second counter-Enlightenment idea is that people are the expendable cells of a superorganism—a clan, tribe, ethnic group, religion, race, class, or nation—and that the supreme good is the glory of this collectivity rather than the well-being of the people who make it up. An obvious example is nationalism, in which the superorganism is the nation-state, namely an ethnic group with a government. We see the clash between nationalism and humanism in morbid patriotic slogans.
>
> (*EN*: 30–31)

For Pinker, a major resistance to liberal universality and reason is the way people desire to be part of a larger group, which often results in a form of nationalism.[52] However, there is a great difference between the idealization of one's nation and the insistence on tradition and social unity. As Freud stresses in *Totem and Taboo*, the central function of every society is to regulate sex and violence, and this regulation results in the introjection of moral distinctions through the formation of the super-ego.[53] Importantly, for Freud, the internalization of a conscience relies on the identification with an arbitrary and irrational form of regulated violence. From this perspective, morality revolves around the desire for regulation both on an individual and collective level. Moreover, this call for regulation is shaped by the primary processes as symbolic mental representations replace natural urges and reality itself.[54] We can therefore think of tradition as the imposition and internalization of social order through the processes of association, substitution, displacement, projection, and introjection.

Although Pinker ties nationalism to ethnic identity, it should be clear that the key factor for this form of ideology is the idealization of a single power, and in this way, like monotheistic religion and monarchy, the submission to one idea or leader is derived from the desire for salvation.[55] Since people want to be saved by some idealized force, they suspend their own individuality and reason as they internalize the social content of their group.[56] Like the case of hypnosis, one does not only submit to the will of the Other: One also internalizes the Other's super-ego, and through the process of suggestion, the meaning and thoughts of the idealized Other becomes the subject's meanings and thoughts.[57] Here, we find the essence of using hypnosis to recover false memories.[58] Through the process of transference, one becomes vulnerable to introjecting implanted memories, and on a national basis, these implanted memories relate to national myths, traditions, and beliefs.[59] Yet, what is vital to stress is that the submission to the source of the content comes first, and then one internalizes the discourse of the Other.[60]

This theory of hypnosis as it relates to authoritarian ideology and the desire for salvation helps to explain why people who are invested in a particular political ideology will accept whatever they hear on a specific media platform.[61] Since they have transferred responsibility onto this Other, they have given up their own reason and reality testing. In fact, Freud posits that the biggest effect of religion is the suspension of critical thinking.[62] As a form of authoritarianism, nationalism also often relies on this type of transference; however, since Pinker represses psychoanalysis, he is unable to see the relational desires shaping the investment in nationalism:

> Nationalism should not be confused with civic values, public spirit, social responsibility, or cultural pride. Humans are a social species, and the well-being of every individual depends on patterns of cooperation and harmony that span a community. When a "nation" is conceived as a tacit social contract among people sharing a territory, like a condominium association, it is an essential means for advancing its members' flourishing.
>
> (*EN*: 31)

In claiming that humans are a social species, Pinker desires to return to a theory of traditional natural order so that he can explain human desires without referring to the primary processes, transference, or narcissism.[63] Thus, instead of realizing that there is no natural moral order or social instinct, he relies on the center-Right idea that higher powers and natural forces shape our current social institutions.[64] Of course, one of the major problems with this perspective is that it prevents us from realizing that humans have to construct their own social institutions by affirming the necessary but impossible ideals of equality, justice, and truth. In other words, democratic law and modern science seek to discover the truth of reality, yet the only way to approach this truth is by committing to the constructed ideal of neutrality.[65] As an ideal, we can never fully attain pure neutrality, still we continue to strive to reach this goal. Moreover, neutrality is the underlying principle that shapes the scientific method and democratic law.

Center-Right Polarization

While Pinker does at times understand these connections among neutrality, universality, equality, and global progress, he continues to confuse different ideologies with each other:

> Religion and nationalism are signature causes of political conservatism, and continue to affect the fate of billions of people in the countries under their influence. Many left-wing colleagues who learned that I was writing a book on reason and humanism egged me on, relishing the

> prospect of an arsenal of talking points against the right. But not so long ago the left was sympathetic to nationalism when it was fused with Marxist liberation movements. And many on the left encourage identity politicians and social justice warriors who downplay individual rights in favor of equalizing the standing of races, classes, and genders, which they see as being pitted in zero-sum competition.
>
> (*EN*: 31)

The first major problem with this analysis is that it equates conservatives and the Right as it also includes traditional and authoritarian ideologies. In fact, it is this type of description that often presents a reductive polarized perspective.[66] Furthermore, as a form of center-Right discourse, Pinker seeks to demonize Left-wing politics as he blames the battle between different identity groups on the call for accommodation.[67] He also does not distinguish between the Left-wing hysterical desire for relieving suffering with the modern liberal desire for equality.

The reason why Pinker may rely on a polarized perspective as he seeks to reject the Leftist call for accommodation is that he has partially bought into the Right-wing libertarian backlash against the welfare state.[68] In claiming that it is the Left that relies on a zero-sum competition between different identity groups, he may be projecting a Right-wing ideology onto the victims of libertarian desires. After all, it is often people on the Right who attack the welfare state and identity politics because they do not want to pay for helping out disadvantaged groups.[69] By applying an imaginary perspective where either the individual is gaining pleasure and freedom, or the other has access to these impulses, the libertarian Right often implies that minorities are stealing their money, jobs, and enjoyment.[70] Therefore, one of the things that they hate about the Left and the welfare state is that this form of politics seeks to take their resources and spend them on some underserving group.[71]

As part of this backlash against the Left, Pinker reveals how he has internalized a Right-wing perspective on climate change:

> The left tends to be sympathetic to yet another movement that subordinates human interests to a transcendent entity, the ecosystem. The romantic Green movement sees the human capture of energy not as a way of resisting entropy and enhancing human flourishing but as a heinous crime against nature, which will exact a dreadful justice in the form of resource wars, poisoned air and water, and civilization-ending climate change.
>
> (*EN*: 32)

Instead of accepting the truth of climate change, Pinker repeats the libertarian criticism of the Left.[72]Thus, all of his efforts to promote reason and science as the keys to global progress are reversed in this ideological denial of climate science.[73]

While Pinker may see himself as a classic liberal, his take on identity politics and climate change demonstrate that his perspective should be called center-Right. Like so many other people who now claim that they just want to base politics on the facts, and they do not hold any particular ideological biases, what we often find is a repressed identification with libertarian ideology.[74] Yet, we should not simply castigate them for their hypocritical stances; rather, we need to understand how they are trying to reconcile competing human relational desires.

Pinker's attempt to present the philosophy, psychology, and politics of globalism is then harmed by his use of polarization and his repressed investment in Right-wing ideology. For example, in the following passage, he articulates one of the reasons why people often reject his view of global progress:

> Another variety of declinism agonizes about the opposite problem—not that modernity has made life too harsh and dangerous, but that it has made it too pleasant and safe. According to these critics, health, peace, and prosperity are bourgeois diversions from what truly matters in life. In serving up these philistine pleasures, technological capitalism has only damned people to an atomized, conformist, consumerist, materialist, other-directed, rootless, routinized, soul-deadening wilderness. In this absurd existence, people suffer from alienation, angst, anomie, apathy, bad faith, ennui, malaise, and nausea; they are "hollow men eating their naked lunches in the wasteland while waiting for Godot."
>
> (*EN*: 32)

The major problem with this rejection of the rejection of global progress is that the Leftist critics he criticizes are at least partially correct: People do suffer from easy access to pleasure and safety, and it would be wrong to simply dismiss how modern capitalism has both enabled economic progress and a host of mental problems.[75]

As a way of safeguarding capitalism and libertarian ideology against a Leftist critique, Pinker's center-Right perspective pushes him to repress the real negative effects of consumer capitalism and climate change.[76] He is also blind to what makes people conform to social norms on a daily basis. As we learn from the psychology of narcissism and the ideology of the center-Left, people seek to have their moral goodness and competence admired by others so that they can repress their own feelings of guilt, shame, and insecurity.[77] Since they want to have their virtue recognized by others, they have to conform to expected social norms, but they also want to be seen as unique individuals, and so they take on an ironic or contradictory subjectivity.[78] As divided subjects, they have to signal that not only are they good people with good intentions, but they are also taking a distance from their own social performance. In the case of Pinker, he wants to represent himself as being a morally good person as he continues to replicate various destructive Right-wing ideas. For instance, he ties his discourse to global progress and the altruistic saving of others: "Knowledge of science, he argued, was a moral imperative, because it could alleviate suffering on a global scale by curing disease, feeding the hungry, saving the lives of infants and mothers, and allowing women to control their fertility" (*EN*: 34). Although I would agree that science has led to global progress and the saving of lives, it is still essential to recognize the limits of science and the need to appeal to other relational desires. In fact, one of the reasons why people are now turning against science, reason, and democracy is that they have other desires that still remain, and different political ideologies cater to these desires in an extreme way.

Since Pinker wants to idealize science as the only solution to the world's problems, he tends to reject any valid criticisms of scientific discourse and its effects:

> Their methodology for seeking the truth consists not in framing hypotheses and citing evidence but in issuing pronouncements that draw on their breadth of erudition and lifetime habits of reading. Intellectual magazines regularly denounce "scientism," the intrusion of science into the territory of the humanities such as politics and the arts. In many colleges and universities, science is presented not as the pursuit of true explanations but as just another narrative or myth. Science is commonly blamed for racism, imperialism, world wars, and the Holocaust. And it is accused of robbing life of its enchantment and stripping humans of freedom and dignity.
>
> (*EN*: 34)

As a replication of the Right-wing attack on Left-wing academics, Pinker mocks the concern that science can lead to racism, war, and extermination.[79] Due to the fact that he wants to see science as an idealized moral good, he attempts to repress any of its negative effects, and then he turns around and attacks the critics.[80]

As he likes to say, progressives hate progress, but the progressives he is mocking tend to be people on the center-Left who often uses their political critiques in order to signal their virtue and reinforce their ideal egos.[81] Therefore, just like the Right, Pinker tends to equate the Left and the center-Left as he represses his own libertarian attitudes. As we shall see in the next chapter, one of the driving forces behind the misunderstanding of ideologies by Pinker and others is a repression of psychoanalysis through the endorsement of a false form of biological determinism.

Notes

1 Pinker, Steven. *Enlightenment now: The case for reason, science, humanism, and progress*. Penguin, 2018. Hereafter cited as "*EN*" in this chapter.
2 Fukuyama, Francis. "The end of history?" In Richard Betts (ed.), *Conflict after the Cold War*. Routledge, 2015: 16–27.
3 Samuels, Robert, and. "Catharsis: The politics of enjoyment." In Robert Samuels, *Žižek and the rhetorical unconscious: Global politics, philosophy, and subjectivity*. Springer, 2020: 7–31.
4 McDonough, Richard. "The limits of the enlightenment." *Language & Communication* 10.4 (1990): 255–265.
5 Woody, J. Melvin, and James Phillips. "Freud's 'Project for a Scientific Psychology' after 100 years: The unconscious mind in the era of cognitive neuroscience." *Philosophy, Psychiatry, & Psychology* 2.2 (1995): 123–134.
6 Freud, Sigmund. *Group psychology and the analysis of the ego*. Hogarth Press, 1949.
7 Lindsay, Heather Fisher. "Balancing community needs against individual desires." *Florida State University Journal of Land Use and Environmental Law* 10.2 (2018): 6.
8 Patrikios, Stratos. "American Republican religion? Disentangling the causal link between religion and politics in the US." *Political Behavior* 30 (2008): 367–389.
9 Finley, Laura, and Luigi Esposito. "The immigrant as bogeyman: Examining Donald Trump and the right's anti-immigrant, anti-PC rhetoric." *Humanity & Society* 44.2 (2020): 178–197.
10 Hofstadter, Richard. *The paranoid style in American politics*. Vintage, 2012.
11 Freud, Sigmund. "Analysis of a phobia in a five-year-old boy." *Collected papers*. Vol. 3. Basic Books, 1955: 149–289.
12 Freud, Sigmund. *Totem and taboo*. Routledge, 2012.
13 Freud, Sigmund. "Formulations on the two principles of mental functioning." In Riccardo Steiner (ed.), *Unconscious phantasy*. Routledge, 2018: 67–76.
14 Mignolo, Walter D. "Enduring enchantment: Secularism and the epistemic privileges of modernity." In Purushottama Bilimoria and Andrew B. Irvine (eds.), *Postcolonial philosophy of religion*. Springer, 2009: 273–292.
15 Dorter, Kenneth. "Science and religion in Descartes' meditations." *The Thomist: A Speculative Quarterly Review* 37.2 (1973): 313–340.
16 Mirsepassi, Ali. "Religious intellectuals and Western critiques of secular modernity." *Comparative Studies of South Asia, Africa and the Middle East* 26.3 (2006): 416–433.
17 Weingart, Peter, and Lars Guenther. "Science communication and the issue of trust." *Journal of Science communication* 15.5 (2016): C01.
18 Mack, Eric, and Gerald F. Gaus. "Classical liberalism and libertarianism: The liberty tradition." In Gerald F. Gaus and Chandran Kukathas (eds.), *Handbook of political theory*. Sage, 2004: 115–130.
19 Henley, Kenneth. "The impersonal rule of law." *Canadian Journal of Law & Jurisprudence* 5.2 (1992): 299–308.
20 Bloom, Paul. "Empathy and its critics." In Troy DuJardin and M. David Eckel (eds.), *Faith, hope, and love: The theological virtues and their opposites*. Springer, 2022: 177–187.
21 Hasson, Yossi, et al. "Are liberals and conservatives equally motivated to feel empathy toward others?." *Personality and Social Psychology Bulletin* 44.10 (2018): 1449–1459.
22 Wagner, Peter. *Modernity*. Polity, 2012.
23 Freud, Sigmund. *The ego and the id*. Simon and Schuster, 2019.
24 Braithwaite, Richard Bevan. "The nature of believing." *Proceedings of the Aristotelian Society* 33 (1932).

25 Pagden, Anthony. *The Enlightenment: and why it still matters.* Oxford University Press, 2013.
26 Smith, Rogers M. "Lockean liberalism and American constitutionalism in the twenty-first century: The Declaration of Independence or 'America First'?" *American Political Thought* 8.2 (2019): 283–295.
27 Samuels, Robert. "Science and the reality principle." In Robert Samuels, *Freud for the twenty-first century: The science of everyday life.* Palgrave Macmillan, 2019: 5–16.
28 Mahmood, Saba. "Secularism, sovereignty, and religious difference: A global genealogy?." *Environment and Planning D: Society and Space* 35.2 (2017): 197–209.
29 Schorske, Carl E. "Freud: The psycho-archeology of civilizations." *Proceedings of the Massachusetts Historical Society* 92 (1980).
30 Freud, Sigmund. *Psychopathology of everyday life.* WW Norton & Company, 1966.
31 Freud, Sigmund. "Repression." *The Psychoanalytic Review (1913–1957)* 9 (1922): 444.
32 Mirvish, Adrian. "Freud contra Sartre: Repression or self-deception?" *Journal of the British Society for Phenomenology* 21.3 (1990): 216–233.
33 Samuels, Robert. "Beyond Hillary Clinton: Obsessional narcissism and the failure of the liberal class." In Robert Samuels, *Psychoanalyzing the Left and Right after Donald Trump: Conservatism, liberalism, and neoliberal populisms.* Springer, 2016: 31–59.
34 Samuels, Robert. *The psychoanalytic understanding of consciousness, free will, language, and reason: What makes us human?.* Routledge, 2023.
35 Lewontin, Richard C., Steven Rose, and Leon J. Kamin. *Not in our genes.* Pantheon Books, 1984.
36 Róheim, Géza. "Animism and religion." *The Psychoanalytic Quarterly* 1.1 (1932): 59–112.
37 Deer, Jemma. "Hatching: Psychoanalysis and the textual unconscious." Jemma Deer, *Radical animism: Reading for the end of the world.* Bloomsbury, 2020: 143.
38 Knight, Robert P. "Introjection, projection and identification." *The Psychoanalytic Quarterly* 9.3 (1940): 334–341.
39 Brunner, José. "Freud and the rule of law: From *Totem and Taboo* to psychoanalytic jurisprudence." *Analytic Freud.* Routledge, 2002: 277–293.
40 Ogden, Thomas H. "On three forms of thinking: Magical thinking, dream thinking, and transformative thinking." *The Psychoanalytic Quarterly* 79.2 (2010): 317–347.
41 Thompson, Michael J. "A functionalist theory of social domination." *Journal of Political Power* 6.2 (2013): 179–199.
42 Moser, Franz. "Beyond Sigmund Freud's *Totem and Taboo* vision for the future-the omnipotence of thought." *International Journal of Foresight and Innovation Policy* 13.3–4 (2018): 187–194.
43 Girard, René. *The scapegoat.* JHU Press, 1989.
44 Compton, Allan. "The psychoanalytic view of phobias: Part I: Freud's theories of phobias and anxiety." *The Psychoanalytic Quarterly* 61.2 (1992): 206–229.
45 Horkheimer, Max, Theodor W. Adorno, and Gunzelin Noeri. *Dialectic of enlightenment.* Stanford University Press, 2002.
46 Westphal, Kenneth R. "Enlightenment, reason and universalism: Kant's Critical Insights." *Studies in East European Thought* 68 (2016): 127–148.
47 Wood, Ellen Meiksins. "Capitalism or enlightenment?." *History of Political Thought* 21.3 (2000): 405–426.
48 Downing, Christine. "Sigmund Freud and the Greek mythological tradition." *Journal of the American academy of religion* 43.1 (1975): 3–14.

49 Freud, Sigmund. *Moses and monotheism*. Sanzani Edizioni, 2023.
50 Samuels, Robert. "Understanding the psychopathology of political ideologies." *Psychoanalysis, Culture & Society* 28.2 (2023): 315–323.
51 Kaplan, Michael. "The rhetoric of hegemony: Laclau, radical democracy, and the rule of tropes." *Philosophy & Rhetoric*43.3 (2010): 253–283.
52 Searle-White, Joshua. *The psychology of nationalism*. Springer, 2001.
53 Kroeber, Alfred Louis. "*Totem and Taboo*: An ethnologic psychoanalysis." *American anthropologist* 22.1 (1920): 48–55.
54 DiCenso, James J. "*Totem and Taboo* and the constitutive function of symbolic forms." *Journal of the American Academy of Religion* 64.3 (1996): 557–574.
55 Riesebrodt, Martin. *The promise of salvation: A theory of religion*. University of Chicago Press, 2010.
56 Spruiell, Vann. "Freud's concepts of idealization." *Journal of the American Psychoanalytic Association* 27.4 (1979): 777–791.
57 McDougall, W. M. "Professor Freud's group psychology and his theory of suggestion." In C. MacFie Campbell, H.S. Langfeld, W. M. McDougall, A. A. Roback, and E. W. Taylor, *Problems of personality*. Routledge, 2013: 267–285.
58 Lynn, Steven Jay. "Informed consent and uninformed clinical practice: Dissociation, hypnosis and false memories." *American Journal of Clinical Hypnosis* 43.3–4 (2001): 311–321.
59 Finlayson, Alan. "Psychology, psychoanalysis and theories of nationalism." *Nations and Nationalism* 4.2 (1998): 145–162.
60 Kunda, Ziva. "The case for motivated reasoning." *Psychological bulletin* 108.3 (1990): 480.
61 Aguado, Jose Fernández. "Psychological manipulation, hypnosis, and suggestion." *International Journal of Cultic Studies* 6 (2015).
62 Gay, Volney. "Sigmund Freud on religion." *Religion, Theory, Critique: Classic and Contemporary Approaches and Methodologies*. Columbia University Press, 2017: 121–126.
63 Swanson, Gillian. "Collectivity, human fulfilment and the 'force of life' Wilfred Trotter's concept of the herd instinct in early 20th-century Britain." *History of the Human Sciences* 27.1 (2014): 21–50.
64 Samuels, Robert. *Psychoanalyzing the politics of the new brain sciences*. Springer, 2017.
65 Zerilli, Linda MG. "This universalism which is not one." *Diacritics* 28.2 (1998): 3–20.
66 Merrill, Samuel, Bernard Grofman, and Thomas L. Brunell. *How polarization begets polarization: Ideological extremism in the US Congress*. Oxford University Press, 2024.
67 Roberts, Jamie Q. *The intellectual dark web: A history (and possible future)*. Pitchstone Publishing, 2025.
68 Doody, Sean. Mapping discourse in the intellectual dark web: A critical computational sociology. Diss. George Mason University, 2022.
69 Rathgeb, Philip, and Marius R. Busemeyer. "How to study the populist radical right and the welfare state?." *West European Politics* 45.1 (2022): 1–23.
70 Salmela, Mikko, and Christian Von Scheve. "Emotional roots of right-wing political populism." *Social Science Information* 56.4 (2017): 567–595.
71 Roper, Kem. From the "war on poverty" to Reagan's "new right," what's in a name?: The symbolic significance of the "welfare queen" in politics and public discourse. Dissertation, University of Louisville, 2012.
72 Samuels, Robert. "The backlash politics of evolutionary psychology: Steven Pinker's blank slate." In Robert Samuels, *Psychoanalyzing the politics of the new brain sciences*. Springer, 2017: 35–58.

73 Galanes, Philip. "The mind meld of Bill Gates and Steven Pinker." *New York Times* 27 (2018).
74 Samuels, Robert. "The centrist history of the culture wars." In Robert Samuels, *Culture wars, universities, and the political unconscious.* Springer, 2024: 15–29.
75 Vijayakumar, Lakshmi, et al. "Suicide in developing countries (2): Risk factors." *Crisis* 26.3 (2005): 112–119.
76 Peters, Michael A. "The enlightenment and its critics." *Educational Philosophy and Theory* 51.9 (2019): 886–894.
77 Samuels, Robert. "Globalization and its discontents: Revisiting the critique of the centrist global elites." In Robert Samuels, *Psychoanalysis and the future of global politics: Overcoming climate change, pandemics, war, and poverty.* Springer, 2023: 73–91.
78 Samuels, Robert. "Ethos, transference, and liberal cynicism." In Robert Samuels, *Žižek and the rhetorical unconscious: Global politics, philosophy, and subjectivity.* Springer, 2020: 49–63.
79 Gudonis, Marius, and Benjamin T. Jones. "Who controls the past?." *History in a post-truth world.* Routledge, 2020: 1–29.
80 Sorell, Tom. *Scientism: Philosophy and the infatuation with science.* Routledge, 2013.
81 Moussaly, Omer. "A historicist critique of Steven Pinker's interpretation of progress." *Dialogue and Universalism* 2 (2021): 285–306.

Chapter 3

Inside the Mind of the Center-Right

Jonathan Haidt and the Naturalization of Ideological Distinctions

In *The Righteous Mind*, Jonathan Haidt does attempt to account for many of the relational desires driving our different ideologies, yet he uses a reductive theory of biological determinism to shape his perspective.[1] Furthermore, similar to Steven Pinker, he reveals an unconscious investment in center-Right politics through the way he defines the different belief systems and political appeals. Moreover, while he does call for the moderation and balancing of distinct ideological demands, his refusal to apply Freudian concepts transforms his discourse into a form of magical thinking and pseudo-science.

The Evolutionary Mind

One of Haidt's major metaphors shaping his work is the notion that we can compare human desires and tendencies to biologically-determined taste buds:

> when you see that some version of kindness, fairness, and loyalty is valued in most cultures, you start wondering if there might be some low-level pan-human social receptors (analogous to taste receptors) that make it particularly easy for people to notice some kinds of social events rather than others.
>
> (*RM*: 142–143)

Thus, in order to account for the apparent universality of certain moral traits and desires, Haidt argues that the moral values of kindness, fairness, and loyalty must be derived from inherited mental programs, which are themselves derived from evolution and the most successful past adaptations.[2] From this perspective, it is not individual experiences that define our core moral tendencies; instead, we are pre-programmed by nature to value certain types of things.

From Haidt's theoretical perspective, our moral values and political ideologies are determined by the interaction between culture and evolution:

DOI: 10.4324/9781003773948-3

> My goal was to find links between virtues and well-established evolutionary theories. I didn't want to make the classic mistake of amateur evolutionary theorists, which is to pick a trait and then ask: "Can I think of a story about how this trait might once have been adaptive?" The answer to that question is almost always yes because reasoning can take you wherever you want to go. Anyone with access to an armchair can sit down and generate what Rudyard Kipling called "just-so stories"—fantastical accounts of how the camel got a hump and the elephant got a trunk. My goal, in contrast, was to identify the most obvious links between two fields I deeply respected: anthropology and evolutionary psychology.
>
> (*RM*: 143–144)

Even though it is important that Haidt does not want to base his analysis on the retroactive use of fictional stories to justify his evolutionary theories, he does still tend to discover an evolutionary cause for current values and beliefs.[3]

Like many evolutionary psychologists and neuroscientist, Haidt often equates minds with brains and humans with other animals:

> Modules are like little switches in the brains of all animals. They are switched on by patterns that were important for survival in a particular ecological niche, and when they detect that pattern, they send out a signal that (eventually) changes the animal's behavior in a way that is (usually) adaptive. For example, many animals react with fear the very first time they see a snake because their brains include neural circuits that function as snake detectors.
>
> (*RM*: 144)

One of the problems with this theory is that people are often afraid of things that do not pose a real risk because their phobias are reliant on the symbolic mental processes of association, substitution, and displacement.[4] Thus, unlike other animals who do not have thought, humans have an imagination that interprets reality in an indirect, irrational, and unintentional manner. While we may be afraid of snakes, many people also fear public speaking or immigrants.[5] It therefore makes little sense to base the conservative desire for protection solely on some type of inherited program dedicated to detecting real threats.

One reason why Haidt wants to turn to evolution and biology to determine relational desires and ideological investments is that he seeks a universal model void of personal and cultural differences:

> This was a perfect description of what universal moral "taste receptors" would look like. They would be adaptations to long-standing threats and opportunities in social life. They would draw people's attention to certain

> kinds of events (such as cruelty or disrespect), and trigger instant intuitive reactions, perhaps even specific emotions (such as sympathy or anger).
> (*RM*: 144)

By basing human emotions and moral intuitions on inherited adaptations, not only is psychology given a biological foundation but so is society.

As I have argued elsewhere, this model of evolutionary determinism is in part based on the repression of the Freudian notions of the drives, the primary processes, the unconscious, transference, and the pleasure principle.[6] By refusing to see how the human mind makes a break with reality, and our drives are not based only on biology, Haidt is able to center ideology on inherited mental programs. However, he is not a strict biological determinist because he also seeks to account for the ways particular cultures help to shape automatic responses:

> This approach was just what we needed to account for cultural learning and variation. Sperber and Hirschfeld distinguished between the original triggers of a module and its current triggers. The original triggers are the set of objects for which the module was designed (that is, the set of all snakes is the original trigger for a snake-detector module). The current triggers are all the things in the world that happen to trigger it (including real snakes, as well as toy snakes, curved sticks, and thick ropes, any of which might give you a scare if you see them in the grass).
> (*RM*: 144–145)

Here through the combination of inherited mental programs, cultural influence, and individual experience, Haidt comes closer to an integrated approach to ideology and psychology, yet he still lacks a full awareness of the effects of mental autonomy and relational desires. Moreover, this integrated theory is often subsumed by a return to evolutionary determinism.[7]

What Haidt and other evolutionary psychologists and neuroscientist do not fully accept is that once they show that cultures and individuals can interpret triggers in diverse and contradictory ways, the role played by biology is greatly diminished:[8]

> Cultural variation in morality can be explained in part by noting that cultures can shrink or expand the current triggers of any module. For example, in the past fifty years people in many Western societies have come to feel compassion in response to many more kinds of animal suffering, and they've come to feel disgust in response to many fewer kinds of sexual activity. The current triggers can change in a single generation, even though it would take many generations for genetic evolution to alter the design of the module and its original triggers.
> (*RM*: 145)

Through this theory of cultural evolution, we are forced to accept the notion that human thought and shared symbolism can overcome any biological programming.[9] Furthermore, what Haidt calls morality, we have called ideology: In other words, what he is really trying to determine is what accounts for the different belief systems, and why do some people identify with one system instead of another?

The Anatomy of Ideologies

Instead of focusing on the core relational desires, Haidt emphasizes what he calls adaptive challenges:

> Five adaptive challenges stood out most clearly: caring for vulnerable children, forming partnerships with non-kin to reap the benefits of reciprocity, forming coalitions to compete with other coalitions, negotiating status hierarchies, and keeping oneself and one's kin free from parasites and pathogens, which spread quickly when people live in close proximity to each other.
>
> (*RM*: 146–147)

Haidt subsequently mentions a sixth adaptive challenge, which he summarizes as "liberty/oppression." By articulating six distinct adaptive challenges, Haidt develops his theory of six major ideologies.[10] According to this theory, what determines someone's ideological beliefs is the way they respond to particular human challenges, like caring for children and forming social partnerships for protection. However, as Freud insists, there is no evidence that we are driven by a biological drive to be social, and so the formation of culture, language, and collective institutions must be tied to the combination of human free will and our ability to imagine things that do not exist in nature or reality.[11]

The main difference between my theory of eight ideologies and Haidt's conception of six moralities is that I do not tie these belief systems to biological adaptations. Thus, while he sees the need to care for children as an inherited program, I argue that this form of social interaction is based on the combination of a fundamental human relationship coupled with an unconscious human desire.[12] While in my theory, the main human desires are for salvation (authoritarian), admiration (center-Left), order (center-Right) protection (conservative), accommodation (Left), liberation (Right), and truth and equality (liberal), Haidt's six moral taste buds are care, fairness, loyalty, authority, sanctity, and liberty/oppression. Moreover, traditional ideology is unintentional, and so while it may be driven by a desire for satisfaction, it can end up in a call for self-punishment.

One of the things that is underlying Haidt choice of moral categories is that most of them can be traced to the current political coalition among authoritarians, traditionalists, libertarians, and conservatives.[13] Furthermore, as we shall see, his definitions and distinctions undermine psychoanalysis and promote a false form of evolutionary psychology. Also, even though he does call for a balancing and moderation of each of these core moralities, he tends to provide a naïve understanding of how they actually affect the world today.

In looking at Haidt's main theoretical matrix, we see how he attempts to combine together cultural and biological evolution:

> ancestors faced these challenges for hundreds of thousands of years, then natural selection would favor those whose cognitive modules helped them to get things right—rapidly and intuitively—compared to those who had to rely upon their general intelligence (the rider) to solve recurrent problems. The second row gives the original triggers—that is, the sorts of social patterns that such a module should detect. (Note that the foundations are really sets of modules that work together to meet the adaptive challenge.) The third row lists examples of the current triggers—the sorts of things that do in fact trigger the relevant modules (sometimes by mistake) for people in a modern Western society. The fourth row lists some emotions that are part of the output of each foundation, at least when the foundation is activated very strongly. The fifth row lists some of the virtue words that we use to talk about people who trigger a particular moral "taste" in our minds.
>
> (*RM*: 147)

The first step in the development of this model is to argue that humans face the same type of challenges throughout history, and within very different cultures, and so the people who survive are the ones who are best able to resolve these core problems. Moreover, since people inherit the solutions that worked in the past, the best responses are the ones that are intuitive and automatic and not the result of intelligence.[14] Here, we see how subjectivity is excluded as people are determined by inherited, automatic programs that are also shaped by particular cultures.

Even though Haidt appears to remove human intelligence from his system, he does argue that the mental programs derived from natural selection can be triggered by unnatural causes due to cultural influences.[15] For instance, while we once had a reason to be afraid of certain things in the distant past, our fear is now triggered by new and different things. Furthermore, the result of this triggering is the production of emotions and not abstract thinking or reason, and these emotions are given particular names in specific cultures.

To help clarify how misguided Haidt's approach turns out to be, we can look at a specific example of the way he defines the morality of care:

> For now, I just want to demonstrate the theory using the Care/harm foundation. Imagine that your four-year-old son is taken to the hospital

> to have his appendix removed. You are allowed to watch the procedure from behind a glass window. Your son is given a general anesthetic and you see him lying, unconscious, on the operating table. Next, you see the surgeon's knife puncture his abdomen. Would you feel a wave of relief, knowing that he is finally getting an operation that will save his life? Or would you feel pain so strongly that you'd have to look away? If your "dolors" (pains) outweigh your "hedons" (pleasures), then your reaction is irrational, from a utilitarian point of view, but it makes perfect sense as the output of a module. We respond emotionally to signs of violence or suffering, particularly when a child is involved, particularly our own child.
>
> (*RM*: 147–148)

In this description of the care/harm module, we find what I would call the hysterical Leftist relation between the innocent victim and the call for accommodation.[16] As Haidt argues, the generation of empathy for the less fortunate depends in part on the notion that only the innocent and the helpless should be cared for.[17] However, what Haidt does not discuss is how we determine if someone is innocent and helpless. In fact, it turns out that a key political issue concerns who is deserving of help from others, and this judgment of who should gain special attention and accommodation is a central aspect of most Left-wing social movements and ideologies and most Right-wing reactions.[18]

Although Haidt wants to base the care/harm response on an inherited mental program, it should be clear that this type of relational desire is derived from cultural and personal interpretations of who is a victim and who is worthy of care.[19] Moreover, as we learn from Freud's theory of hysteria, people often use real and imagined suffering in order to manipulate others and to gain a sense of identity on an unconscious level.[20] Yet, this type of unconsciousness is not caused by inherited programs; instead, for Freud, the unconscious is derived from repression, and repression is based on the use of self-deception in order to protect one's self-image.[21]

In the case of individual hysteria, we often stigmatize the person who fakes an illness or constantly complains, but in the realm of politics, the presentation of suffering can trigger positive social change.[22] As a mode of protest, the display of suffering makes a call for accommodation, and we can trace the foundations of the modern welfare state to this hysterical structure.[23] However, as many people on the Right often point out, it is possible for some people to not really deserve help, especially if they are not really innocent, helpless victims.[24] My main point here is that Haidt's conception of the morality of harm/care is not only reductive and misguided, but it also leaves out the essential role that subjectivity and interpretation play in morality and ideology.

In the summary of his five moral categories, Haidt reveals many of the ideological distortions inherent in his theory of ideology: "The five rows illustrate violations of Care (hurting a child), Fairness (profiting from someone else's undeserved loss), Loyalty (criticizing your nation to outsiders), Authority (disrespecting your father), and Sanctity (acting in a degrading or disgusting way)" (*RM*: 152). One problem with this list is that all of the examples can be associated with your typical Republican voter who believes that it is wrong to hurt children and that one should reject outsiders and respect fathers and sacred objects. In other words, there is an unconscious ideological bias that shapes his theory of ideology.[25]

The Evolution and Psychology of Care

Returning to the morality of care, Haidt articulates the origins of this moral taste bud based on a theory of evolutionary adaptation:

> Mammals make fewer bets and invest a lot more in each one, so mammals face the challenge of caring for and nurturing their children for a long time. Primate moms place even fewer bets and invest still more in each one. And human babies, whose brains are so enormous that a child must be pushed out through the birth canal a year before he or she can walk, are bets so huge that a woman can't even put her chips on the table by herself. She needs help in the last months of pregnancy, help to deliver the baby, and help to feed and care for the child for years after the birth. Given this big wager, there is an enormous adaptive challenge: to care for the vulnerable and expensive child, keep it safe, keep it alive, keep it from harm.
>
> (*RM*: 153–154)

I would argue that by tracing the harm/care module to the relation between the caring mother and the helpless child, Haidt both expresses and represses Freud's theory of the cause for transference, idealization, and authoritarian ideology.[26] From the psychoanalytic perspective, when the suffering baby cries and the parent acts to make the suffering go away, the parent is placed in a position of idealized power where responsibility is shifted from the subject to the Other. On one level, it is correct to say that the first step is the expressed suffering of the child (hysteria), but the second step relies on a mental trick where accommodation is turned into a call for salvation.[27] The child then not only wants to get special attention for its suffering: It also turns the Other into an idealized savior. In contrast, with hysteria, the Other is usually demonized as the one who has harmed the subject and who deserves retribution by the innocent victim.[28]

The main issue then is not how much investment the mother has put into raising the helpless child: The real issue is how the child interprets the role of the parent and other potential helpers. Thus, we know that children growing up in the same family can have very different psychologies and ideologies, and one of the main causes for these differences has to do with how they have interpreted their fundamental relationships.[29] Clearly, biological evolution is not the most important factor in tracing the origins of a particular person's morality and ideology.

Since Haidt believes in a mixture of biological determinism and cultural evolution, he wants to argue that the Care/Harm module also helps to define why people care for others who belong to the same group:

> And it's not only mothers who need innate knowledge. Given the number of people who pool their resources to bet on each child, evolution favored women and (to a lesser extent) men who had an automatic reaction to signs of need or suffering, such as crying, from children in their midst (who, in ancient times, were likely to be kin). The suffering of your own children is the original trigger of one of the key modules of the Care foundation.
>
> (*RM*: 154–155)

While Freud also argues that the original relation with a caregiver expands to other social relationships, he distinguishes between salvation and accommodation, and one of the main differences is that salvation requires the idealization of the Other and the effacement of the self.[30] As a key aspect of authoritarian ideology, this mode of transference represents a radical break with nature and evolution since one has to take a leap of faith by believing that only the Other knows and cares.

The Authoritarian Other

It should be noted that by capitalizing the word Other, I am referring to Hegel, Lacan, and Sartre who all point to the way that humans tend to create a generalized mental category of people and things that have great power and influence.[31] For instance, in religious belief, one treats God as the one who knows and controls everything, and in therapy, it is often the therapist who is placed in this idealized position.[32] Interestingly, what Haidt tends to leave out of his discussions of care, loyalty, authority, and sanctity are the destructive aspects of these types of relationships. In contrast, Freud tends to only focus on the negative aspects as he sees all authoritarian relationships as mainly based on a loss of individual reason and reality testing.[33] Yet, if we tie the idealization of authority to the desire for salvation based on caregiving, then we should realize that some level of care and trust is necessary for all humans.

As Haidt himself realizes, the question of who deserves our help has changed over time as different categories of people are considered to be innocent victims of harm: "The current triggers can change rapidly. We care about violence toward many more classes of victims today than our grandparents did in their time" (*RM*: 156). This theory helps us to understand why we need Leftist social movements to expand who is considered to be worthy of universal equality and protection, yet this process is undermined when groups become fixated on their own suffering and their need for special accommodation (equity).[34] In fact, the conflict between the Leftist call for equity and the liberal demand for equality has often undermined the solidarity of progressive political movements.[35]

Liberal or Libertarian?

For Haidt, modern liberal democracy is driven by the fairness module, yet his conception of fairness feeds into a libertarian fear of being cheated by undeserving others:

> The original triggers of the Fairness modules are acts of cooperation or selfishness that people show toward us. We feel pleasure, liking, and friendship when people show signs that they can be trusted to reciprocate. We feel anger, contempt, and even sometimes disgust when people try to cheat us or take advantage of us.
>
> (*RM*: 159)

On the one hand, Haidt is correct in relating the liberal call for fairness to the way children want to make sure that others are not given an unfair advantage.[36] However, a key to modern liberal democracy is the transformation of this relational desire to the ideal of universality.[37] By embodying this call for universality in the institutions of science and democratic law, a global system of reason and equality can be instituted; however, this form of universality is not part of nature or evolution: It is a human social construct that needs to be protected in order to be maintained.[38] Meanwhile, the fear of being cheated by others relates to the libertarian desire to have total access to freedom and pleasure without having to sacrifice for society.[39]

Instead of clearly distinguishing between the Leftist call for accommodation and the liberal goal of universality, Haidt combines the two under the category of fairness:

> On the left, concerns about equality and social justice are based in part on the Fairness foundation—wealthy and powerful groups are accused of gaining by exploiting those at the bottom while not paying their "fair share" of the tax burden.
>
> (*RM*: 159–160)

While the goal of many on the Left may be to have a more equal society, the clear opposition between the victimized minority and the oppressive Other relates to a hysterical fantasy of victimization structured by a binary splitting between the innocent self and the evil Other.[40] It is this type of structure and pathology that enables the disempowered to call for accommodation as they seek a remedy for their suffering.

Interestingly, Haidt claims that everyone wants fairness; although, the Right and the Left have a different view of this relational desire: "Everyone cares about fairness, but there are two major kinds. On the left, fairness often implies equality, but on the right it means proportionality—people should be rewarded in proportion to what they contribute, even if that guarantees unequal outcomes" (*RM*: 160–161). In the presentation of this false equivalence between the Right and the Left, Haidt confuses the liberal ideal of equality with the Leftist demand for equity and the Right-wing acceptance of inequality. It is therefore hard to comprehend how his discourse, then, leads to a clearer understanding of ideological differences. In fact, what tends to motivate his center-Right position is his desire to demonize the Left and give a free pass to the Right.[41]

Naturalizing Loyalty

Another way that he distorts ideological distinctions is through his conception of the desire for loyalty:

> The male mind appears to be innately tribal—that is, structured in advance of experience so that boys and men enjoy doing the sorts of things that lead to group cohesion and success in conflicts between groups (including warfare). The virtue of loyalty matters a great deal to both sexes, though the objects of loyalty tend to be teams and coalitions for boys, in contrast to two-person relationships for girls.
>
> (*RM*: 162)

This imposition of a gender opposition reflects the way the center-Right often relies on the activation of a traditional social hierarchy and culture in order to rationalize the dominance of men in contemporary society.[42] In other words, by implying that there is a natural order shaping the traditional social hierarchy, Haidt naturalizes a socially constructed gender distinction.

For Haidt, the loyalty module entails that there has always been war, group rivalry, and coalitions:

> And it now appears that warfare has been a constant feature of human life since long before agriculture and private property. For millions of years, therefore, our ancestors faced the adaptive challenge of forming and maintaining coalitions that could fend off challenges and attacks from rival groups.
>
> (*RM*: 163)

Since he sees male dominance and competition as natural and inevitable, he equates the traditional social order privileging men over women with an automatic, inherited, adaptive program.[43] However, as Freud stresses, what really helps to rationalize and justify male dominance is the belief in a symbolic order and hierarchy based on binary oppositions combined with the primary processes of projection and introjection.[44] From this perspective, individuals confuse symbolic representations with the perception of reality as they also treat external cultural hierarchies as the result of their own thinking.[45]

Through the process of introjection, culture is internalized, and then through projection, it is naturalized, yet for Haidt, it is nature itself that is driving cultural representations and the symbolic social order:

> The Loyalty/betrayal foundation is just a part of our innate preparation for meeting the adaptive challenge of forming cohesive coalitions. The original trigger for the Loyalty foundation is anything that tells you who is a team player and who is a traitor, particularly when your team is fighting with other teams. But because we love tribalism so much, we seek out ways to form groups and teams that can compete just for the fun of competing. Much of the psychology of sports is about expanding the current triggers of the Loyalty foundation so that people can have the pleasures of binding themselves together to pursue harmless trophies. (A trophy is evidence of victory. The urge to take trophies—including body parts from slain foes—is widespread in warfare, occurring even during modern times.).
>
> (*RM*: 163)

According to the theory of evolutionary psychology, the drive for loyalty and social organization is derived from the way that collective action is able to protect against external and internal threats, and since this mode of coalition building was successful in the past, it has been internalized as an automatic biological intuition.[46]

One of the problems with this turn to evolutionary psychology to explain current ideologies is that it relies on naturalizing social structures that are often formed through violence and magical thinking.[47] Moreover, as Haidt's own example above reveals, the traditional imposition of morality is being confused with the phobic conservative focus on protecting against imagined threats. Perhaps the biggest problem with his approach to the morality of loyalty is that he does not separate the call for social regulation from the submission to an idealized single authority:

> The love of loyal teammates is matched by a corresponding hatred of traitors, who are usually considered to be far worse than enemies. The Koran, for example, is full of warnings about the duplicity of out-group members, particularly Jews, yet the Koran does not command Muslims to kill Jews. Far worse than a Jew is an apostate—a Muslim who has

> betrayed or simply abandoned the faith. The Koran commands Muslims to kill apostates, and Allah himself promises that he "shall certainly roast them at a Fire; as often as their skins are wholly burned, We shall give them in exchange other skins, that they may taste the chastisement."
>
> (*RM*: 164)

On the one hand, it is evident that traditional cultures make a clear distinction between the in-group and external enemies, yet on the other hand, what helps to define monotheistic religions is the centralization of power coupled with a loss of reality testing by the members of the group. In this mode of authoritarian ideology, the belief in the One who will save the true believers represents a transformation of the traditional call for social regulation.[48]

As Haidt insists, this moral emphasis on complete loyalty also shapes the foundation of nationalism:

> The left tends toward universalism and away from nationalism, so it often has trouble connecting to voters who rely on the Loyalty foundation. Indeed, because of its strong reliance upon the Care foundation, American liberals are often hostile to American foreign policy.
>
> (*RM*: 164)

The first thing to remark about this passage is that Haidt equates liberals and the Left as he posits that the reason why Democrats lose elections is that they do not promote a nationalistic approach to foreign policy.[49] Thus, instead of catering to the desire for authoritarian submission, the liberals and the Left are criticized for not supporting their team in a loyal way. Part of what is missing in this faulty argument is the way nationalism combines traditional social order with authoritarian submission and the centrist desire for admiration.[50] Since some Americans want to believe that their team is the best, and it is always innocent, they treat the nation as an extension of their own idealized ego.[51] Thus by idealizing the nation, they can also idealize themselves, and this narcissistic call for admiration helps to repress any guilt and shame that can be associated with the state.[52]

Authoritarian Ideology

In turning to the morality of authoritarianism, Haidt attaches this ideology to the natural world and the actions of other animals:

> The obvious way to begin thinking about the evolution of the Authority foundation is to consider the pecking orders and dominance hierarchies of chickens, dogs, chimpanzees, and so many other species that live in groups. The displays made by low-ranking individuals are often similar across species because their function is always the same—to appear

> submissive, which means small and nonthreatening. The failure to detect signs of dominance and then to respond accordingly often results in a beating.
>
> (*RM*: 166)

Although it is true that other animals also have a form of social hierarchy, it should be clear that mental thought and complex language separate humans from these other beings, and in the case of authoritarian ideology, the key distinction is the way humans have a desire to transfer responsibility to an idealize Other who is supposed to provide salvation.[53] Moreover, by pointing to the use of violence in the animal world to instill social order, Haidt once again naturalizes human social constructs.[54] In other words, his own center-Right discourse is a form of animism where cultural formations are equated with a natural order, and by confusing thoughts with reality, he seeks to lend credibility to his imaginary interpretations.[55]

While humans rely on others to help them survive, and this dependency can result in a mode of authoritarian idealization, other animals do not structure their worlds through the use of thoughts and symbols.[56] Yet, in Haidt's description of the origin of authoritarianism, he returns to animals as the source for this belief system:

> So far this doesn't sound like a promising origin story for a "moral" foundation; it sounds like the origin of oppression of the weak by the powerful. But authority should not be confused with power. Even among chimpanzees, where dominance hierarchies are indeed about raw power and the ability to inflict violence, the alpha male performs some socially beneficial functions, such as taking on the "control role." He resolves some disputes and suppresses much of the violent conflict that erupts when there is no clear alpha male. As the primatologist Frans de Waal puts it: "Without agreement on rank and a certain respect for authority there can be no great sensitivity to social rules, as anyone who has tried to teach simple house rules to a cat will agree."
>
> (*RM*: 166)

One problem with this theory is that humans are not cats or chimps, and so their relation to authority and groups needs to be distinguished from the way other animals act. Since we have the ability to imagine things that do exist, and we are not determined by our instincts, humans have relational desires shaped by symbolic representations.[57] Furthermore, it is strange that Haidt wants to separate authority from power since one of the main functions of authoritarian ideology is to justify the centralization of power within a society or group.

From Freud's perspective, it is essential to distinguish monotheistic religions from traditional animistic cultures because what is key to the transition from animism to monotheism is the way that a desire for salvation centralizes power and authority.[58] Thus, while monotheistic religions do utilize many of the rituals, beliefs, and practices of traditional cultures, the defining move is to base authority and loyalty on the idealization of the One who can save each individual and society itself.[59] Even though this moral desire is derived from the way that caregivers help to alleviate the suffering of the child, this call for help is transformed into the total submission to the will of the Other.

As Freud highlights, "primitive" traditional cultures often believed in multiple gods, and since they denied the reality of death, they thought that when someone dies, their spirit returns and often makes people feel guilty and afraid.[60] In this structure, the spirit of the dead Other acts as an externalized super-ego, which itself is the projection of an introjected cultural morality.[61] With the transition from animism to monotheism, there is the added focus on single source of authority and control, which Haidt partially recognizes in the following passage:

> This control role is quite visible in human tribes and early civilizations. Many of the earliest legal texts begin by grounding the king's rule in divine choice, and then they dedicate the king's authority to providing order and justice. The very first sentence of the Code of Hammurabi (eighteenth century BCE) includes this clause: "Then Anu and Bel [two gods] called by name me, Hammurabi, the exalted prince, who feared God, to bring about the rule of righteousness in the land, to destroy the wicked and the evil-doers; so that the strong should not harm the weak."
> (*RM*: 166–167)

Clearly, this theory that the king's authority is derived from God's will represents a major aspect of monotheistic religions and the establishment of premodern monarchies.

As Haidt indicates, all of the moral attitudes contain both a positive and negative side since their origins are shaped by basic human relational desires, but what turns these moral demands into ideological fixations is the way that a single relational desire becomes extreme and dominates the other moral claims:

> Human authority, then, is not just raw power backed by the threat of force. Human authorities take on responsibility for maintaining order and justice. Of course, authorities often exploit their subordinates for their own benefit while believing they are perfectly just.
> (*RM*: 167)

As we see with the formation of cults, the desire for order, protection, and salvation can result in the idealization of someone who exploits people for their own benefit. The danger, then, of authoritarian ideology is that it combines blind submission with the justification of the power, greed, and manipulation of a sociopathic leader.[62]

Haidt explains that as a good liberal, he first believed that hierarchy equates to power, exploitation, and evil, yet he soon learned that he was wrong:

> Fiske's theory of the four basic kinds of social relationships includes one called "Authority Ranking." Drawing on his own fieldwork in Africa, Fiske showed that people who relate to each other in this way have mutual expectations that are more like those of a parent and child than those of a dictator and fearful underlings: In Authority Ranking, people have asymmetric positions in a linear hierarchy in which subordinates defer, respect, and (perhaps) obey, while superiors take precedence and take pastoral responsibility for subordinates. Examples are military hierarchies … ancestor worship ([including] offerings of filial piety and expectations of protection and enforcement of norms), [and] monotheistic religious moralities … Authority Ranking relationships are based on perceptions of legitimate asymmetries, not coercive power; they are not inherently exploitative.
>
> (*RM*: 167–168)

In this idealization of authoritarianism, Haidt follows Freud in basing this type of relationship on a repetition of the relation between a child and a parent; however, what he does not fully realize is that this fundamental relational desire can be easily exploited by people with power.[63] Similar to Aristotle's justification of slavery, Haidt implies that people want to submit to authority because it provides social order and protection in a mutually beneficial manner.[64]

The Return of the Center-Right

As I have been arguing, this combination of traditional, conservative, and authoritarian ideologies represents a central aspect of the current Republican Party in the United States and other authoritarian movements around the world; meanwhile, this desire to accept social authority is often combined today with the opposite desire, which is for individual freedom (libertarianism).[65] In this structure, the desire for salvation, protection, and symbolic order serve to enhance and protect the desire of individuals who want to use their authority and privilege to exploit others and not share their wealth with the less fortunate. From this perspective, the idealization of authority serves as a cover for the justification of inequality and exploitation.[66] Haidt unintentionally feeds this authoritarian ideology when he rationalizes and naturalizes social authority: "If authority is in part about protecting order and fending off chaos, then everyone has a stake in supporting the existing order and in holding people accountable for fulfilling the obligations of their station" (*RM*: 168). By appealing to the desires for protection, order, and authority, Haidt ends up repressing the roles that violence, exploitation, and abuse play in contemporary authoritarian ideology: "As with the Loyalty foundation, it is much easier for the political right to build on this foundation than it is for the left, which often defines itself in part by its opposition to hierarchy, inequality, and power" (*RM*: 168). What Haidt appears to be saying here is that the reason why Democrats lose elections is that they fail to emphasize loyalty to authority because they desire to have a more equal and just society. In other words, he has internalized the Right-wing attack on the Left, the center-Left, and liberalism as he seeks to hide his ideology under the cover of a fake scientific discourse.

We can consider Haidt's turn to evolutionary theory to explain current ideological formations as a conspiracy theory dedicated to imposing a false sense of order and causality by imagining a hidden power that secretly controls everything.[67] In turn, this theory allows him to appear to be scientific and rational while he uses the manipulation of traditional cultural beliefs in order to provide a totalizing perspective. What then makes his discourse a product of the center-Right is that his commitment to selfish greed and the exploitation of others is hidden by his self-representation of being unbiased and objective.

As we shall see in the next chapter, Haidt's employment of evolutionary psychology and neuroscience can also result in a center-Left mode of academic discourse and narcissism. What these two ideological positions share in common is that they both try to hide their own biases under a false sense of scientific neutrality. Moreover, while the center-Right is driven by a desire to justify inequality, the center-Left is driven by a desire for admiration.

Notes

1 Haidt, Jonathan. *The righteous mind: Why good people are divided by politics and religion*. Vintage, 2012. Hereafter cited as "*RM*" in this chapter.

2 Samuels, Robert. "The backlash politics of evolutionary psychology: Steven Pinker's blank slate." In Robert Samuels, *Psychoanalyzing the politics of the new brain sciences*. Springer, 2017: 35–58.

3 Haidt, Jonathan. "The new synthesis in moral psychology." *Science* 316.5827 (2007): 998–1002.

4 Freud, Sigmund. *Obsessions and phobias*. Read Books, 2014.

5 Starkstein, Sergio. "Sigmund Freud and the psychoanalytical concept of fear and anxiety." In Sergio Starkstein, *A conceptual and therapeutic analysis of fear*. Springer, 2018: 231–257.

6 Samuels, Robert. *The psychoanalytic understanding of consciousness, free will, language, and reason: What makes us human?*. Routledge, 2023.

7 Saltzstein, Herbert D., and Tziporah Kasachkoff. "Haidt's moral intuitionist theory: A psychological and philosophical critique." *Review of General Psychology* 8.4 (2004): 273–282.

8 Samuels, Robert. "The brain sciences against the welfare state." In Robert Samuels, *Psychoanalyzing the politics of the new brain sciences.* Springer, 2017: 85–114.
9 Henrich, Joseph, and Richard McElreath. "The evolution of cultural evolution." *Evolutionary Anthropology: Issues, News, and Reviews* 12.3 (2003): 123–135.
10 Haidt, Jonathan, Jesse Graham, and Craig Joseph. "Above and below left–right: Ideological narratives and moral foundations." *Psychological Inquiry* 20.2–3 (2009): 110–119.
11 Greisman, Harvey C. "Herd instinct and the foundations of biosociology." *Journal of the History of the Behavioral Sciences* 15.4 (1979): 357–369.
12 Samuels, Robert. "Freud's Project." In Robert Samuels, *(Mis)understanding Freud with Lacan, Žižek, and neuroscience.* Springer, 2022: 7–28.
13 Blum, Lawrence. "Political identity and moral education: A response to Jonathan Haidt's The Righteous Mind." *Journal of Moral Education* 42.3 (2013): 298–315.
14 Saltzstein, Herbert D., and Tziporah Kasachkoff. "Haidt's moral intuitionist theory: A psychological and philosophical critique." *Review of General Psychology* 8.4 (2004): 273–282.
15 Jonason, Peter K., and David P. Schmitt. "Quantifying common criticisms of evolutionary psychology." *Evolutionary Psychological Science* 2.3 (2016): 177–188.
16 Samuels, Robert, and Robert Samuels. "Pathos, hysteria, and the Left." In Robert Samuels, *Žižek and the rhetorical unconscious: Global politics, philosophy, and subjectivity.* Springer, 2020: 33–47.
17 Cole, Alyson Manda. *The cult of true victimhood: From the war on welfare to the war on terror.* Stanford University Press, 2007.
18 Petersen, Michael Bang, et al. "Who deserves help? Evolutionary psychology, social emotions, and public opinion about welfare." *Political Psychology* 33.3 (2012): 395–418.
19 Samuels, Robert. "The brain sciences against the welfare state." In Robert Samuels, *Psychoanalyzing the politics of the new brain sciences.* Springer, 2017: 85–114.
20 Freud, Sigmund. *Dora: An analysis of a case of hysteria.* Simon and Schuster, 1997.
21 Menaker, Esther. "The self-image as defense and resistance." *The Psychoanalytic Quarterly* 29.1 (1960): 72–81.
22 Hoffman, Martin L. "Empathy, justice, and social change." In Martin L. Hoffman, *Empathy and moral development: Implications for caring and justice.* Cambridge University Press, 2014: 71–96.
23 Feldman, Stanley, et al. "The interplay of empathy and individualism in support for social welfare policies." *Political Psychology* 41.2 (2020): 343–362.
24 Zwolinski, Matt. "Libertarianism and the welfare state." In Jason Brennan, Bas van der Vossen, and David Schmidtz (eds.), *The Routledge handbook of libertarianism.* Routledge, 2017: 323–341.
25 Haidt, Jonathan, and Jesse Graham. "When morality opposes justice: Conservatives have moral intuitions that liberals may not recognize." *Social Justice Research* 20.1 (2007): 98–116.
26 Freud, Sigmund. "Project for a scientific psychology." In James Strachey (ed.), *The standard edition of the complete psychological works of Sigmund Freud.* Vol. 1. Hogarth Press, 1953–1974: 283–397.
27 Perlman, Eleanore Armstrong. "Introduction: Narcissism and object choice in Freud." *British Journal of Psychotherapy* 3.1 (1986): 60–64.
28 Freud, Sigmund. *The ego and the id.* Simon and Schuster, 2019.
29 Schafer, Roy. "The loving and beloved superego in Freud's structural theory." *The Psychoanalytic Study of the Child* 15.1 (1960): 163–188.
30 Freud, Sigmund. *Moses and monotheism.* Sanzani Edizioni, 2023.

31 Anderson, Pamela Sue. *The Other*. Oxford University Press, 2013.
32 Eizirik, Cláudio Laks. "Freud's group psychology, psychoanalysis, and culture." In Ethel Spector Person (ed.), *On Freud's "Group psychology and the analysis of the ego"*. Routledge, 2018: 155–173.
33 Coyle, Robert Burns. *A comparison of authoritarian and permissive techniques used in hypnosis*. Ball State University, 1982.
34 Samuels, Robert. "Pathos, hysteria, and the Left." In Robert Samuels, *Žižek and the rhetorical unconscious: Global politics, philosophy, and subjectivity*. Springer, 2020: 33–47.
35 Minow, Martha. "Equality vs. equity." *American Journal of Law and Equality* 1 (2021): 167–193.
36 Cooper, David E. "Equality and envy." *Journal of Philosophy of Education* 16.1 (1982): 35–47.
37 Hendershott, Anne. *The politics of envy*. Sophia Institute Press, 2020.
38 Franks, Bradley. "Social construction, evolution and cultural universals." *Culture & Psychology* 20.3 (2014): 416–439.
39 Samuels, Robert. "Catharsis: The politics of enjoyment." In Robert Samuels, *Žižek and the rhetorical unconscious: Global politics, philosophy, and subjectivity*. Springer, 2020: 7–31.
40 Samuels, Robert. "Pathos, hysteria, and the Left." In Robert Samuels, *Žižek and the rhetorical unconscious: Global politics, philosophy, and subjectivity*. Springer, 2020: 33–47.
41 Keckler, Charles, and Mark J. Rozell. "The libertarian right and the religious right." *Perspectives on Political Science* 44.2 (2015): 92–99.
42 Chalmers, Jocelyn, et al. "The Rights of Man: Libertarian Concern for Men's, But Not Women's, Reproductive Autonomy." *Political Psychology* 44.3 (2023): 603–625.
43 Christmas, William. "Libertarianism and privilege." *Molinari Review* 1.1 (2016).
44 Staiger, Janet. "Taboos and totems: Cultural meanings of *The Silence of the Lambs*." In Jim Collins, Ava Preacher Collins, and Hilary Radner (eds.), Film theory goes to the movies: Cultural analysis of contemporary film. Routledge, 1993: 142–154.
45 Levine, Michael G. "The subject is taboo." *MLN* 101.5 (1986): 977–1002.
46 Van Vugt, Mark, and Mark Schaller. "Evolutionary approaches to group dynamics: An introduction." *Group Dynamics: Theory, Research, and Practice* 12.1 (2008): 1.
47 Lewontin, Richard C., Steven Rose, and Leon J. Kamin. *Not in our genes*. Pantheon Books, 1984.
48 Assmann, Jan, et al. *Freud and monotheism: Moses and the violent origins of religion*. Fordham University Press, 2018.
49 Williams, Colin. "Nationalism in a democratic context." In John Agnew, Katharyne Mitchell, and Gerard Toal (eds.), *A companion to political geography*. Wiley, 2003: 356–377.
50 Finlayson, Alan. "Psychology, psychoanalysis and theories of nationalism." *Nations and Nationalism* 4.2 (1998): 145–162.
51 Voigt, Katrin. "Nationalism as collective narcissism: the pathology of an everyday practice." *Journal of Psychosocial Studies* 17.3 (2024): 238–250.
52 Loewenberg, Peter. "The psychodynamics of nationalism." *History of European Ideas* 15.1–3 (1992): 93–103.
53 García-García, Juan. "A neglected legacy: Massenpsychologie und ich-analyse in the era of nations and nationalism." *Psychotherapy and Politics International* 19.3 (2021): e1603.

54 Hakokōngäs, Juho Eemeli, and Inari Hannele Sakki. "The naturalized nation: Anchoring, objectification and naturalized social representations of history." *Journal of Social and Political psychology* 4.2 (2016): 646–669.
55 Viriasova, Inna. "Biopolitics and community of life: Between naturalism and animism." *Parrhesia: A Journal of Critical Philosophy* 22 (2015): 90–105.
56 Viriasova, Inna. "Biopolitics and community of life: Between naturalism and animism." *Parrhesia: A Journal of Critical Philosophy* 22 (2015): 90–105.
57 Samuels, Robert. "Neuroscience and the repression of psychoanalysis." In Robert Samuels, *(Mis)understanding Freud with Lacan, Žižek, and neuroscience.* Springer, 2022: 29–62.
58 Holt, Robert R. "On Freud's authoritarianism." *The Psychoanalytic Review* 102.3 (2015): 315–346.
59 Friedman, R. Z. "Freud's religion: Oedipus and Moses." *Religious studies* 34.2 (1998): 135–149.
60 Róheim, Géza. "Animism and religion." *The Psychoanalytic Quarterly* 1.1 (1932): 59–112.
61 Freud, S. "Libidinal types." *The Psychoanalytic Review (1913–1957)* 26 (1939): 438.
62 Henderson, Jennifer. Psychological manipulation and cluster-B personality traits of cult leaders. Diss. Walden University, 2023.
63 Kriegman, Daniel, and Leonard Solomon. "Cult groups and the narcissistic personality: The offer to heal defects in the self." *International Journal of Group Psychotherapy* 35.2 (1985): 239–261.
64 Garnsey, Peter. *Ideas of slavery from Aristotle to Augustine.* Cambridge University Press, 1996.
65 Ray, John J. "Libertarians and the authoritarian personality." *The Journal of Libertarian Studies* 4.1 (1980): 39–43.
66 Havercroft, Jonathan, and Justin Murphy. "Is the tea party libertarian, authoritarian, or something else?." *Social Science Quarterly* 99.3 (2018): 1021–1037.
67 Katyal, Neal Kumar. "Conspiracy theory." *Yale Law Jounal* 112 (2002): 1307.

Chapter 4

Critiquing the Ideological Brain

This chapter offers a critique of the turn to biology in order to understand ideology. By providing a close reading of Leor Zmigrod's *The Ideological Brain*, I offer an alternative, integrated theory of human relational desires.[1] Moreover, through a return to Freud's fundamental work on social formations, I reveal how a center-Left mode of analysis presents a fake form of liberal, scientific thinking. As we shall see, a repressed polarized perspective shapes this discourse on an unconscious and narcissistic level.

Introducing the Ideological Brain

At the start of her book, Zmigrod makes the strong claim that our brains are driven to understand the world and develop a sense of belonging to a social community: "Our brain—an organ that constantly seeks to understand the world around us, to feel belonging with others—is delighted by our newfound ideological possessions" (*IB*: 2). The first thing to stress here is that she is not focusing on the human mind; instead, she seeks to tie our search for meaning and belonging to the biological brain, and by replacing the mind with the brain, she is able to repress the fundamental theories of psychoanalysis.[2] Moreover, her discourse is structured by a desire to make her work appear more scientific than it actually may be.[3]

One way of understanding this move to biological determinism is to relate it to the narcissistic desire for admiration.[4] Although it appears that she just wants to be more rational and therefore liberal, the key difference between the center-Left and modern liberal science is that the center-Left is driven by a relational desire for admiration as one seeks to have the good self recognized by others.[5] In fact, the main way that she signals her virtue is by idealizing her own claim to mental openness, which is opposed by her to the of rigidity of ideology. As the joke goes, there are two type of people, those who believe that there are two types of people, and those who do not. In Zmigrod's case, she tends to divide people between those who have a rigid approach to the world and those who are more open and flexible, and as she will make clear in her work, she belongs to the latter group.

DOI: 10.4324/9781003773948-4

Through her use of brain imaging research and other neuroscientific techniques and theories, Zmigrod follows the current fad of pretending that we can explain mental experiences by tracing them back to inherited mental programs derived from natural selection and localized in particular brain regions.[6] Furthermore, she resolves the difficult problem of consciousness by replacing psychological experiences with physical structures. From a Freudian perspective, we can understand this move as relating to how consciousness itself is often shaped by the primary processes that treat words as if they were things and things as if they were words.[7] Moreover, what we find in this new form animism is that culture and psychology are given a false material foundation by substituting the brain for the mind:

> I studied what brains look like when they obey commands as opposed to when they form free and spontaneous decisions. With the techniques of neuroscience, I learned that obedient actions evoked neural activity patterns that were markedly different from free choices.
>
> (*IB*: 2)

The irony of this approach is that at the very moment Zmigrod celebrates the need to be free, open, and avoid rigidity, she presents a very rigid theory and interpretation of ideology and human psychology.

What is so fascinating about this critique of ideological rigidity is the way it demonstrates unknowingly how someone can be completely unaware of their own rigidity as they present a false sense of being open and rational.[8] Here we encounter ideology functioning on an unconscious level because the perspective that frames one's thoughts and perceptions is itself repressed and hidden by a desire to present a positive self-image.[9] Since Zmigrod wants to see herself as one who is open and rational and not rigid or dogmatic, she has to hide from herself her own rigidity. Furthermore, as the following statement reveals, part of this process relates to repressing the unconscious itself: "Under the glow of pixelated neural impulses, I searched for the subterranean, unconscious markers of human freedom" (*IB*: 3). Like many other neuroscientists and evolutionary psychology, Zmigrod equates the unconscious with hidden mental processes, but as Freud stresses, the unconscious is not defined by what we do not know; rather, the unconscious is the result of repression, and repression is caused by self-deception, which itself serves the function of protecting one's idealized self-image.[10]

The Irony of the Center-Left

What we often find in narcissistic personalities is that one wants to think that one is free and unique at the very moment one is conforming to the expectations of others.[11] Since the driving force of narcissism and the center-Left is to be admired by others due to one's moral goodness and exceptionality, there is a fundamental conflict that cannot be resolved: After all, how can one be admired for one's conformity to social expectations and at the same time be recognized for one's individuality and specialness?[12]

I argue that this tension between conforming and being exceptional structures the psychopathology of center-Left ideology, which often dominates in education and progressive politics.[13] As we learn from Matthew Stewart's *The 9.9%*, the psychology of upper-middle class professionals is often shaped by the need to signal one's moral virtue as one also engages in anti-social drives for power, privilege, profit, and prestige.[14] In fact, what people often don't like about the educational elite is that they seem hypocritical because they pretend to care about social equality, while they take advantage of inequality.[15] For instance, even though the majority of faculty at American universities and colleges now suffer from low wages and a lack of shared governance, the tenured professors want to see themselves as being good people committed to equality and democracy.[16] Moreover, the way that one gets admiration and a promotion is by conforming to the norms of one's discipline as one also attempts to show how one's contributions are unique and special.[17]

In Zmigrod's case, it is clear that she wants to make her discourse conform to the social expectations of her academic field through her use of established concepts and theories, and yet she also wants to claim that she is free from the reductive application of rigid definitions and interpretations as she makes an original contribution to the field:

> George Orwell observed that "political language ... is designed to make lies sound truthful and murder respectable, and to give an appearance of solidity to pure wind." We assign people and ideas into neat categories in the pursuit of clarity and identity.
>
> (*IB*: 11)

While Zmigrod is clearly critical of the application of neat categories in the pursuit of clarity and identity, her own discourse is dominated by this use of binary oppositions in order to provide the appearance of being scientific and true.[18]

In a very telling passage, she reveals how rigid linguistic concepts and definitions can act to repress our messy thoughts, feelings, and desires:

> Yet these linguistic buckets mask the realities of ideologies as they are lived—messily, hypocritically, proudly, self-destructively—with loss, joy, humor, regret, fear, reversals, retractions, ruminations, intimacy, and grief—with tears and lamentations, beaming smiles, and confused sideways glances.
>
> (*IB*: 11)

In other words, the application of rigid oppositions and concepts not only shape our perceptions, but they also act to deceive us about our own subjectivity.[19] For Zmigrod, this use of predetermined mental constructs defines the essence of all ideologies:

> Despite the complexities and contradictions, there are commonalities in how ideologies are practiced and preached, regardless of their aims or their claims. Whether nationalist or racist or religious, there are parallels in how all ideologies infiltrate human minds. These resemblances are not coincidences; they are inherent to the structure of ideological thinking.
> (*IB*: 11)

The major problem with this theory is that it fails to focus on the distinctions among different ideologies as it concentrates on the rigid binary opposition of rigidity and flexibility. Moreover, by positing that a flexible mind is one that avoids all ideology, she falls into the trap of clearing a space for an idealized non-ideological perspective.[20]

Interestingly, even though she tends to equate ideology with mental rigidity, she also realizes that ideologies can themselves be flexible and changing:

> Ideologies are sold to us as timeless and fixed, but they are in fact highly fluid and mobile. These clusters of ideas are perpetually changing, taking on novel guises in every generation. Ideological worldviews can switch sides and policy preferences. Parties of tradition campaign for radical reform while progressive movements hesitate to innovate.
> (*IB*: 10)

As we shall see, this claim that ideologies only appear to be rigid contradicts her main argument concerning the connection between ideology and mental rigidity.

One reason why she contradicts herself concerning the flexibility of ideologies is that she tends to treat all ideologies as if they are derived from the same type of thinking: "As the political thinker Eric Hoffer observed in *The True Believer*, 'there is a certain uniformity in all types of dedication, of faith, of pursuit of power, of unity and of self-sacrifice'" (*IB*: 11). The only way that she is able to argue that all ideologies are shaped by the same mental tendencies is by not seeing how each ideology relates to a very specific relational desire.[21] For example, the traditional imposition of morality and social order is very different from the authoritarian desire for salvation and the libertarian pursuit of freedom. When we fail to make these distinctions, we lose our ability to understand various ideologies and psychopathologies.

Distinguishing Ideologies

While part of her theory attempts to derive ideology from inherited brain functions, the other part relies on a more cultural and psychological perspective:

> In its simplest formulation, an ideology is a kind of narrative. A compelling story about the world. Yet not all stories are ideologies, and not all forms of collective storytelling are rigid and oppressive. There is a difference between culture and ideology. Ideologies offer absolutist descriptions of the world and accompanying prescriptions for how we ought to think, act, and interact with others. Ideologies legislate what is permissible and what is forbidden. Unlike culture—which can celebrate eccentricities and reinterpretations—in ideology, nonconformity is intolerable and total alignment is essential. When deviation from the rules leads to severe punishment and ostracism, we have moved away from culture and into ideology.
>
> (*IB*: 11–12)

This desire for a narrative can be related to the traditional imposition of order since stories act to provide a sense of certainty through the use of the symbolic primary processes of association, substitution, and displacement.[22] One way then of understanding traditional culture is that it allows for predictability in a chaotic world, and yet Zmigrod wants to distinguish between culture and ideology so that she can tie ideology to rigidity.

I believe that an important theoretical mistake she makes is that she confuses intensity with quality by arguing that any belief system becomes ideological when it becomes extreme or rigid.[23] The reason, then, why she does not differentiate among distinct ideologies is that she is not really interested in the particular content of each belief system; instead, she wants to focus on the intensity of the commitment:

> From fascism and communism to eco-activism and spiritual evangelism, ideological groups offer absolute and utopian answers to societal troubles, strict rules for behavior, and an ingroup mentality through dedicated practices and symbols. These features exist across the spectrum of ideological persuasions. Such characteristics can emerge even when the ideology is guided by the sincerest intentions and noblest ideals—even if it claims to protect human dignity or flourishing.
>
> (*IB*: 12)

Here we see what happens when one does not clearly separate the eight major ideologies from each other: The result is that one gains a sense of clarity and certainty; however, this attitude simply represents the over-generalization of traditional ideology.[24]

While it is true that many different belief systems do rely on the primary processes that shape traditional ideology, each perspective relies on a distinct relational desire. For instance, religious fundamentalists may seek order and meaning through narratives, yet this traditional desire is coupled with an emphasis on the desire to be saved by the idealized Other.[25] In turn, even though libertarians may use stories and lies to justify their actions, they are driven by a desire for individual freedom to act on their impulses and emotions without restriction.[26] Likewise, the center-Left ideology may produce a rigid psychology through the unconscious use of primary processes, but the main relational desire is for admiration in order to prove to the self that it is good and special.[27]

Since Zmigrod refuses to separate the different belief systems and relational desires, she tends to see every ideology through the lens of traditional belief systems:

> As though from the heavens, these -isms describe the contours of life and prescribe human action, instructing us about the cosmos and how we ought to relate to others within it. For believers, the utopian destiny of an ideology seems carved from the clouds of eternity. A looming force soaring above our heads, meant to be venerated and revered.
>
> (*IB*: 12)

This notion that all ideologies describe and prescribe human actions points to the ways traditional belief systems are based on a symbolic regulation of social actors.[28]

For Zmigrod, what defines ideology is a form of rigid thinking and not a particular relational desire or belief system: "Individual minds convert social doctrines into ideological thinking, a style of thinking that is governed by strict mental rules and carefully regimented mental leaps" (*IB*: 12). By focusing on the rigidity of a specific way of thinking, she seeks to separate the study of ideology from history and particular social movements: "While most definitions perceive ideologies as historical currents and sociological movements, I am interested in examining ideologies as psychological phenomena instead" (*IB*: 12). In this decontextualized approach, what really matters is if people think in a rigid or open way: "Does the ideology impose a tight grip on believers' brains? Or does it let them wonder and wander freely?" (*IB*: 13). The end result of her project, then, is to reduce the study of ideology to an analysis of the binary opposition between open and closed thinking.

As a mode of splitting and polarization, Zmigrod's research is structured by not only a rigid opposition but also a clear moral distinction:

> When an ideology demands rigid and ritualistic thinking, it demands that we bias our vision, twist our gnawing doubts into silence, surrender our subjectivities and creative possibilities. When an ideology demands rigid and ritualistic thinking, it demands that we become someone else. Someone less singular and unique, less curious, less free.
>
> (*IB*: 13)

Since she clearly values being curious and free, her analysis is structured by a particular moral hierarchy structured through its own rigid, reductive lens.[29]

Moreover, her emphasis on free thought may indicate an unacknowledged investment in a libertarian ideology dedicated to the freedom of the individual who is not constrained by social restrictions.[30]

The Ideology of Fake Science

Zmigrod's valorization of individualism and personal liberty is associated with her use of neuroscience in order to concentrate on the individual brain instead of the collective dimensions of ideology: "I hope to show that we can challenge ideologies on different terms—on the terms of the single individual. The individual brain" (*IB*: 13). It should be clear that the analysis of an individual's brain could act to hide the social and collective aspects of culture and ideology.[31] While my theory focuses on relational desires, her approach relates to the mental processes of isolated brains. Furthermore, we know that people often do not know all of the mental content associated with the shared ideologies they internalize.[32]

For Zmigrod, mental rigidity defines ideology, and this way of thinking is opposed to the more open and flexible form of thought that she endorses:

> If we have less scope for plasticity and change and less direct access to our sensations, we are at risk of dehumanizing ourselves and others. We become less sensitive, less elastic, less authentic. If we see reality through an ideological lens, we end up avoiding the richness of existence in favor of a more reduced, stereotyped experience. By studying the ideological brain with neuroimaging devices and cognitive tests, we can illuminate previously invisible forms of domination. With the tools of science, we can develop new ways to critique ideologies.
>
> (*IB*: 13–14)

Here we see how her own rigid binary logic is applied at the very moment she critiques rigid analysis. Furthermore, her discourse seeks to find credibility and valorization by being attached to the science of neuroimaging, which itself has often been disputed.[33]

By relying on the reductive opposition of rigidity versus flexibility, she shapes her scientific discourse in a rigid way: "A science of ideology can inspire us to question our idols, our icons, our metaphors, our imagined utopias. It can stimulate careful analysis and honest self-reflection. It can even become the basis for personal or social action" (*IB*: 14). This critique of metaphors is itself ironic since her entire approach relies on the metaphorical substitution of brains for minds.[34] However, due the fact that she does not appear to be aware of her own reductive filter and metaphorical representations, we can consider her rhetoric as blocking the type of honest self-reflection she desires to celebrate.

Although it may appear that I simply picking on this particular writer, much of her work is indicative of how the new brain sciences are seeking to replace the social sciences and psychoanalysis with an unaware pseudo-science.[35] In fact, the reason why many of the new brain sciences should be considered to be pseudo-sciences is that they rely on the rigid imposition of symbolic metaphors without taking into account how these substitutions distort reality and understanding. We can see some of the effects of this approach in the following passage:

> Believing passionately in a rigid doctrine is a process that spills into our neurons, flowing into our bodies. Ideologies are not mere envelopes for our lives; they enter our skins, our skulls, our nerve cells. Totalizing ideologies shape the brain as a whole, not simply the brain when it is confronted with political propositions or debates. Science is beginning to reveal that the profound reverberations of ideologies can be observed in the brain even when we are not engaging with politics at all.
>
> (*IB*: 14)

The first move here is to eliminate the distinction between ideological ideas and the physical structures of the brain. Even though external social representations can act to reshape parts of our internal mental structures, it is misleading to say that ideology inhabits our neurons or enters our skin.[36] Here we are witnessing the metaphorical confusion of minds and bodies as the psychological is projected onto the material world, and just as in animism, thoughts are treated as if they were actualized in external reality.

A key delusion structuring this work, then, is the notion that there is no real differences among the social, the biological, and the psychological:

> Since our brains learn to embody indoctrination in deep and insidious ways, the social rituals we learn to enact can become the biological realities of our minds and bodies. There is therefore a danger that when an individual is immersed in rigid ideologies, it is not only their political opinions and moral tastes that are being sculpted—their entire brain is being sculpted too.
>
> (*IB*: 14)

By equating the mind, society, and the body, her rigid binary framing is coupled with a unifying rhetoric that acts to erase essential conceptual differences.[37]

Zmigrod not only uses brain mapping to detect the inner-workings of society and individual psychology, but she also presents a series of experiments that all tend to conflate natural reflexes with internalized social content and routinized behavior:

> This is where I step out of the experiment and tell you that your natural reaction to the change can tell me almost everything about you. Your

> spontaneous response to the fact that the old rule stopped working and you needed to discover a new one to survive is a kind of inadvertent confession. In this simple game of stars and circles, you have accidentally and inevitably exposed your innermost beliefs.
>
> (*IB*: 18–19)

In this passage, one's inner-most beliefs and thoughts are equated with natural reactions as if there is no difference between nature and human psychology.[38]

On the most basic level, Zmigrod uses her experiments in order to show that people who have a fast and rigid response to unexpected stimuli also display a rigid commitment to ideologies:

> What I, the experimenter, the scientist, have discovered is that how you perform in this game can give me clues about your whole approach to life. Your level of rigidity in this neuropsychological test foreshadows the rigidity with which you believe in ideologies in the social and political world. Your perceptual reflexes are linked to your ideological reflexes.
>
> (*IB*: 20)

By equating perception with ideological commitment, she leaps over the great divides between minds and bodies and individuals and society: Of course, what allows her to make these moves is her reliance on the metaphorical substitution of brains for minds and her refusal to clearly separate biology, psychology, and culture.[39]

If we try to understand why she imposes such a rigid and reductive frame, we have to acknowledge that not only does it feed the traditional desire for symbolic order, but it also represents a desire for admiration as she uses her pseudo-science to idealize her own self-image as being open and flexible, which from her perspective defines modern liberal ideology:

> When my colleagues and I invited thousands of people to complete cognitive tests of mental flexibility such as this game, called the Wisconsin Card Sorting Test, we found that the people who are the most behaviorally adaptable on neuropsychological tasks are the same people who—in the realm of ideologies—are most open-minded, most accepting of plurality and difference.
>
> (*IB*: 20)

What these experiments really show is that it does not matter how much one conforms to the formal processes of scientific experimentation if one frames one's perceptions through the lens of misguided concepts and definitions.[40] As much as Zmigrod would like to pretend that she is not only open-minded but also empirical, her own approach tells a much different story.

Like many other center-Left false liberals, Zmigrod appears to be driven by a strong desire to signal her willingness to tolerate opposing ideas:

> The people with the most flexible minds are the people who acknowledge that the intellectual realm can be separated from the personal realm. They do not viscerally hate their interlocuters—they may hate their opinions but they do not project that hatred onto the persons voicing them. (*IB*: 20)

What I think she is endorsing here is the notion that true liberals are for open debate and are flexible enough not to take the arguments of their oppositions to heart.[41] As we have seen in recent culture wars, this valorization of free speech, debate, and the diversity of viewpoints may appear to be a product of liberal ideology, modern science, and democracy, yet it is often used to legitimate intolerant, Right-wing hate speech.[42]

It is telling that at the moment she wants to promote mental and cultural flexibility, she returns to the rigid, reductive notion that biology and thought are really the same thing because they both entail information processing:

> When neuroscientists talk about cognition and perception, we are talking about information processing that deals with simple stimuli, with basic sensory information in neutral contexts. Cognitive tasks are composed of uncomplicated elements—colored shapes and moving black dots—displayed on spare, undecorated screens. Through these tasks, we are not assessing how you deal with emotionally evocative or triggering information—information that genuinely scares you or makes you feel a sour pinch of disgust. We are not studying tasks that are too cognitively demanding or complex—ones that would exasperate you needlessly. When neuroscientists measure cognition and perception, we glean individual differences in how a brain forms decisions, learns from the environment, and responds to challenges or contradictions at the most foundational level. (*IB*: 20–21)

By equating minds and brains based on the concept of information processing, Zmigrod opens the door for also considering nature and the mind as computers preprogrammed by evolution.[43] However, there is a world of difference between perception and cognition just as there is a profound distinction between human thought and computers.

Repressing Freud

In a very telling moment, Zmigrod shows how unlike computers and other animals, humans can deceive themselves about their own thoughts and feelings:

> These individual differences are implicit; we have little conscious access to them or control over their expression. A cognitively rigid person may insist that they are spectacularly flexible, and an adaptable thinker may believe that they lack mental malleability. It is astonishing how rarely we know ourselves.
>
> (*IB*: 21)

This lack of self-awareness is what Freud calls the unconscious, and the cause for this mental state is repression, which is itself a form of self-deception relying on self-division.[44] Ironically, Zmigrod's own work is a great example of this type of mental contradiction because she presents herself as being flexible and open while she applies a very rigid framework in an unaware way. Moreover, since she represses psychoanalysis itself, she does not account for the differences between the mind and the body, the individual and society, and consciousness and the unconscious.[45]

Similar to other neuroscientists and evolutionary psychologists, Zmigrod confuses a lack of conscious awareness with the psychoanalytic notion of the unconscious:

> The ideological brain's rigidities and idiosyncrasies manifest where we least expect them, in our most private sensations and physiological responses, beneath the surface of our public convictions and conscious feelings. The dangers of dogmatic ideologies are therefore not just political—the consequences are neural, individual, and existential.
>
> (*IB*: 21)

In saying that ideology shapes our neurons in a hidden way, Zmigrod returns to a biological version of the mind and culture itself while she also replaces attention to the content of belief systems with the level of commitment to them.[46]

One of the effects of Zmigrod's approach is that she appears to mock the idea that the internet or charismatic leaders can implant ideological content into the minds of individuals:

> If we conceive of the mind as a container to be emptied or to be filled, someone else is doing the emptying and the filling up. The believer's mind is not complicit or responsible. Harmful ideas have been tipped into it by an external force—The internet! Those shady friends! That charismatic preacher! The victim is not at fault. They are under occupation.
>
> (*IB*: 23)

Since she is interested in the form of thought and not its content, she ignores the Freudian notion that the hypnotist, leader, or lover can suggest ideas that are soon internalized by the submissive follower.[47]

However, at the same time that Zmigrod downplays the source and content of ideology, she also states that symbolic thinking feeds our desire for meaning and order:

> Metaphors are powerful because they have the flavor of explanations. But an analogy taken too literally becomes a source of error and confusion. In fact, a metaphor mistaken for the truth is worse than an error: it reinforces certain superstitions and faulty excuses. A wrong metaphor discounts behavior that ought to be scrutinized and changed.
>
> (*IB*: 24)

This recognition of the power of metaphorical thinking is akin to Freud's notion of the symbolic primary processes where unrelated things are equated through the processes of mental and linguistic association, substitution, and displacement.[48] Yet, what Zmigrod does not herself admit is that her entire project is itself centered on the metaphorical substitution of the brain for the mind.

In pointing to the role of rhetoric in structuring our perceptions, she highlights how all ideologies begin with the human tendency to mistake symbolic representations for reality:

> As the linguists George Lakoff and Mark Johnson wrote in their influential study of metaphors, *Metaphors We Live By*, "metaphors may create realities for us, especially social realities. A metaphor may thus be a guide for future action. Such actions will, of course, fit the metaphor. This will, in turn, reinforce the power of the metaphor to make experience coherent. In this sense metaphors can be self-fulfilling prophecies."
>
> (*IB*: 24)

As the foundation of animism and traditional ideology, metaphorical thinking points to the relational desire for order where it does not exist in reality.[49] What the infant then wants from its hallucinations and the "primitive" culture wants from its rituals is the same basic human desire for symbolic repetition.[50] Therefore, in the cause of hallucination, Freud posits that when a child is missing the desired object, the first response is to imagine the repetition of a previous scene of satisfaction.[51] Likewise, when an animistic culture imagines that the spirit of a dead person has come back to haunt people, they are not only projecting their super-ego in a psychotic way onto reality, but they are also repeating earlier experiences in a symbolic form.[52]

Transference and Authoritarian Ideology

Instead of fully grasping this underlying psychotic core of traditional belief systems, Zmigrod focuses on critiquing the notion that particular situations can cause people to adopt rigid ideologies:

> Situational explanations assume that, under the right—or wrong—conditions, we are all potential tyrants. And if we are all the same, all at fault by virtue of an inherent wickedness of the human heart, then none of us is responsible. Conformity and obedience become impossible to resist. Failures of moral conduct hinge on strong situations, insane situations, acute situations, in which all of us would become divorced from ourselves and capable of committing acts of cruelty.
>
> (*IB*: 25)

While Zmigrod appears to dismiss this theory of social psychology based on the way particular situations make people prone to succumb to rigid ideologies, Freud's theory of transference affirms that specific types of social relationships—like those presented in hypnosis, passionate love, the church, the army, and political rallies—allow for someone to suspend their own critical thinking and reality testing as they submit to the will of the Other, which also results in a process of suggestion.[53]

It is vital to stress that transference can lead to an authoritarian relationship, which may also utilize traditional content. However, Freud is clear to differentiate between the primary processes of an animistic belief system and the centralized authority we find in monotheism and other premodern forms of submission.[54] In fact, the social psychologists that Zmigrod appears to dismiss all echo Freud's fundamental insight into how certain social situations can trigger radical conformity:

> In the 1950s and 1960s, social psychologists became infatuated with these situational explanations. Famous psychologists placed innocent university students in situations of torture or imprisonment; ridiculous (and recklessly unethical) experiments in which participants were drummed up to obey, conform, and inflict pain on strangers. At Yale, Stanley Milgram encouraged participants to administer electric shocks to their innocent peers—and a majority complied.
>
> (*IB*: 25)

The reason why Zmigrod wants to reject these social theories and experiments is that her argument relies on replacing specific social content and situations with particular styles of thinking located in particular brain processes:

> All these crazed experiments sought to prove that it is the situation, not the person, that mattered. Millions of psychology textbooks have disseminated these results and crowned the conclusions as evidence that we are all prone to conformity. In pressurized situations, we would all obey.
>
> (*IB*: 26)

Clearly, these experiments showed that some people do not obey and conform, and yet Zmigrod misreads the findings so that she can dismiss the entire notion of social influence.[55] However, with Freud's theory of transference-neurosis, we discover that certain people are prone to submit to an idealized Other, and this submission does not rely on any particular psychopathology or style of thinking.[56] In fact, the very process of therapy relies on individuals desiring to be saved by their therapists, and this is both the strength and the danger of transference.[57] Moreover, transference and the desire for salvation define authoritarian ideologies, which may or may not utilize traditional ideological content.

An Ironic Use of the Brain Sciences

Strangely, Zmigrod wants to use the theory of metaphor in order to discredit the role played by transference:

> Metaphors shape the experiments we run, the theories we curate, and ultimately the moral weight with which we judge ourselves and others. If we prioritize the situation as the primary force of ideological action, we neglect individual differences and variation in behavior.
>
> (*IB*: 26)

From this perspective, a reliance on the theory of social conformity negates the ways different individuals react to particular social contexts, yet, this over-emphasis on metaphorical thinking serves to hide the true essence of authoritarian ideologies. Also, while Zmigrod appears to be very sensitive to how metaphorical thinking shapes our perception of reality, she is herself blind to her own use of metaphors.[58]

Since she constantly sees brains as a substitute for minds in order to produce a theory based on natural order, her entire project can be considered to be shaped by metaphor. Yet, she also wants to reject the same theories she constantly utilizes as she questions the power of evolution to shape our minds: "The view of the ideological mind as passive and complacent, at the mercy of uncontrollable forces or evolutionary norms, is both pessimistic and wrong. In fact, the 'mindless mind' is an oxymoron: What mind can be empty of itself?" (*IB*: 27). What Zmigrod does not realize is that she herself has emptied the mind by replacing it with the brain, but in her efforts to make her discourse sound scientific, she has to both employ and reject the theory of evolutionary determinism.[59]

This use and repression of biological determinism is a common feature in evolutionary psychology and neuroscience where we often find a desire to both point to an underlying natural order and the possibility of social influence through the concept of plasticity.[60] The problem with this strategy is that it is structured by a contradictory combination of rigidity and flexibility:

After all, one cannot say that the locus of ideology is in the individual brain shaped by evolution, while also asserting that the human mind is open and flexible. In fact, what in part allows for this contradiction is the imaginary overcoming of the separation between the mind and the body:

> Many of these metaphors of the mind as a container—whether full of misinformation or empty of substance—reflect an outdated assumption that thoughts are nonphysical, immaterial. This assumption is called dualism, and it implies that brains and bodies are made of different and separable substances. The body as physical and tangible and the mind as nonphysical and spiritual. Subscribers to dualism believe that the stuff in our heads—our thoughts, our mind, our personality—is fundamentally different from the stuff that constitutes our bodies—organic matter governed by chemistry and physics.
>
> (*IB*: 27)

Similar to Haidt's notion of "moral taste buds," Zmigrod's conception of the ideological brain seeks to overcome the distinction between the mental and the physical though the use of a metaphorical substitution where biology replaces psychology, and yet what distinguishes humans from other animals is our ability to imagine things that do not exist in reality.[61] For Freud, the primary processes enable hallucinations, dreams, and superstitions, which allows for reality to be replaced by symbolic representations, yet neuroscientists and evolutionary psychologists usually cannot accept this separation between the spiritual mind and the physical brain.[62]

Often in these discourses, we find a misunderstanding of Descartes and his conception of the relation between thinking and material reality:

> Descartes was in a bind. Either render the soul a matter of physics and let psychology flow from physiology (and with it, renounce the specialness of the Christian soul), or find a way to uphold the mind–matter distinction and save Christianity from contradiction with reason.
>
> (*IB*: 28)

The way, then, to overcome Cartesian dualism is to simply reject the vital distinction between the mental and the physical.[63] Although Zmigrod is correct to point out that Descartes wants to save both the Christian notion of the soul and the modern ideology of reason and science, what she does not accept is that we have to affirm and separate different mental processes and ideologies. While traditional ideology relies on spirituality and the notion of the mind transcending material reality, the ideology of modern liberalism depends on the necessary but impossible ideals of equality and neutrality.[64]

Descartes argues that we are thinking both when we are awake and when we are dreaming, and thus thought itself must be irrational, indirect, and unintentional, and yet, he also affirms that the key to modern science is to suspend all prejudices and pre-suppositions as we try to see reality in an objective, neutral manner.[65] Descartes adds that reason is equal in all people, and so at the foundations of liberal democracy, we find the ideals of equality and universality. However, even though the goal of reason and science is to verify the truth of external reality, we can only approach this reality by assuming the necessary but impossible ideal position of impersonal neutrality.[66] From this perspective, liberalism is also an ideology because it relies on unnatural ideals implemented on a personal and social basis.

Since Zmigrod does not realize that her own perspective depends on a certain mode of idealism, she tends to critique this way of thinking as itself being ideological: "In these settings there is a disunity between mind and body that ideologies use to keep adherents servile and that encourages followers to commit violence against themselves in the name of a transcendent ideal" (*IB*: 29). One of the problems with this criticism of transcendent ideals is that humans can never escape this way of thinking: The real question should be what type of ideals shape one's perceptions and understanding.

Due to her investment in an anti-Freudian notion of the mind, she obsessively returns to the idea that there is no distinction between the mind and the body or the mind and the brain: "To understand the ideological brain, we must shed these dualistic assumptions. The brain is composed of the same material as the rest of the body—water, protein, fat, salt, blood vessels, tubes, and fibers" (*IB*: 29). This type of argument is similar to saying that there is no distinction between a piano and a song; even though a song can be produced on a piano, songs and pianos belong to very different categories.

For philosophy and neuroscience, the "hard problem" is to determine how we move from a physical structure to a mental experience, and yet she wants to wish away this difficulty through a system of metaphorical substitutions: "Every thought we experience is physical, every emotion is physiological, every dream and conviction is a biological signature produced by the brain and body" (*IB*: 29). It should be clear that thoughts are not physical, and psychology is not biology, but from her perspective, these differences do not matter.[67] Perhaps she wants to eliminate the hard problem of consciousness because she desires to replace thoughts with mechanical processes preprogrammed by evolution: "But the mind-brain distinction can also sustain the illusion that our psychology is imbued with a nonphysical spirituality, something eternal and otherworldly. An essence independent of the body" (*IB*: 29). The problem with this attempt to eliminate spirituality is that it also gets rid of one of the central modes of ideology, which is traditionalism. However, without this desire for mental autonomy over reality, we lose what makes us human and also what enables different ideological belief systems.

I call her approach pseudo-science because it relies on metaphors that are not acknowledged and serve to produce a fake form of evidence and credibility. Although she presents her discourse as purely scientific, it should be evident that it is really based on an unconscious manipulation of language.[68] For instance, instead of affirming the distinction between the mind and the brain, she simply treats them as if they are one through a process of symbolic substitution:

> Here, the boundary between mind and brain is purposefully dissolved. I use mind and brain interchangeably because there is little scientific evidence that a human mind exists that is not a brain. Change the brain—injure it, nurture it, mess with it—and our psychic lives change too.
>
> (*IB*: 29–30)

While it is true that a brain injury can cause a change in mental states, that does not mean that the brain and the mind are the same thing. Moreover, while we may need brains in order to have minds, we also need hardware to have software, and no one would say that they are the same thing.[69]

The Political Body

Ultimately, she makes it clear that the reason why she wants to wish away the difference between the mental and the physical is that she desires to equate the mental with the biological: "I talk of the ideological brain because I want to make it clear that the mental is biological, and the biological is shaped by the political" (*IB*: 30). While the first move here is to replace psychology with biology, the second move is to posit that the political shapes biology. This double movement is similar to Freud's theory of the primary processes and animistic cultures, which are based on both projection and introjection.[70] Thus, in the case of projection, internal mental representations are experienced as being part of the natural world, but with introjection, the external culture is internalized and treated as coming from one's own thoughts.[71] These two movements, then, represent the core of traditional ideology.

To better understand the origins and structures of this desire for natural order and the resultant investment in animism and traditional ideology, the next chapter will examine Aristotle's *Rhetoric*, which represents an idealization and naturalization of social hierarchy. In other words, politics is a seen as a product of nature; however, this form of ideological naturalization is dependent on a narcissistic desire to idealize the self. The reason why it is so important to look at this ancient Greek thinker is that he articulates in a repressed way the connection between conservative, authoritarian, and traditional ideologies from a center-Right perspective.

Notes

1 Zmigrod, Leor. *The ideological brain*. Henry Holt, 2025. Hereafter cited as "*IB*" in this chapter.

2 Samuels, Robert. "Neuroscience and the repression of psychoanalysis." In Robert Samuels, *(Mis)understanding Freud with Lacan, Žižek, and neuroscience*. Springer, 2022: 29–62.
3 Satel, Sally, and Scott O. Lilienfeld. *Brainwashed: The seductive appeal of mindless neuroscience*. Basic Civitas Books, 2013.
4 Baumeister, Roy F., and Kathleen D. Vohs. "Narcissism as addiction to esteem." *Psychological Inquiry* 12.4 (2001): 206–210.
5 Samuels, Robert. "(Liberal) Narcissism." In Yannis Stavrakakis (ed.), *Routledge handbook of psychoanalytic political theory*. Routledge, 2019: 151–161.
6 Legrenzi, Paolo, and Carlo Umiltà. *Neuromania: On the limits of brain science*. Oxford University Press, 2011.
7 Freud, Sigmund. *On dreams*. Courier Corporation, 2012.
8 Uziel, Liad, and Bentzion Cohen. "Self-deception and discrepancies in self-evaluation." *Journal of Research in Personality* 88 (2020): 104008.
9 Berthold, Charles Ernest Whitby. *Narcissism and the regulation of self-esteem through self-deception*. Georgia State University-College of Education, 1991.
10 Joseph, Rhawn. "Awareness, the origin of thought, and the role of conscious self-deception in resistance and repression." *Psychological Reports* 46.3 (1980): 767–781.
11 Samuels, Robert. "Ethos, transference, and liberal cynicism." In Robert Samuels, *Žižek and the rhetorical unconscious: Global politics, philosophy, and subjectivity*. Springer, 2020: 49–63.
12 Magill, R. Jay. *Chic ironic bitterness*. University of Michigan Press, 2009.
13 Samuels, Robert. "Beyond Hillary Clinton: Obsessional narcissism and the failure of the liberal class." In Robert Samuels, *Psychoanalyzing the Left and Right after Donald Trump: Conservatism, liberalism, and neoliberal populisms*. Springer, 2016: 31–59.
14 Stewart, Matthew. *The 9.9 percent: The new aristocracy that is entrenching inequality and warping our culture*. Simon and Schuster, 2022.
15 Hedges, Chris. *Death of the liberal class*. Vintage Canada, 2011.
16 Samuels, Robert. *Educating inequality: Beyond the political myths of higher education and the job market*. Routledge, 2017.
17 Whatley, Mark A., et al. "Understanding academic entitlement: Gender classification, self-esteem, and covert narcissism." *Educational Research Quarterly* 42.3 (2019): 49–70.
18 Elbow, Peter. "The uses of binary thinking." *Journal of Advanced Composition* (1993): 51–78.
19 Wood, Jack Denfeld, and Gianpiero Petriglieri. "Transcending polarization: Beyond binary thinking." *Transactional Analysis Journal* 35.1 (2005): 31–39.
20 Gross, Alan G. "The roles of rhetoric in the public understanding of science." *Public Understanding of Science* 3.1 (1994): 3.
21 Samuels, Robert. *The psychopathology of political ideologies*. Routledge, 2021.
22 Freud, Sigmund. *Totem and taboo*. Routledge, 2012.
23 Lewins, Frank. "Recasting the concept of ideology: A content approach." *The British Journal of Sociology* 40.4 (1989): 678–693.
24 Lazere, Donald, and Anne-Marie Womack. "Overgeneralization, stereotyping, and prejudice." In Donald Lazere and Anne-Marie Womack, *Reading and writing for civic literacy*. Routledge, 2017: 183–203.
25 Riesebrodt, Martin. "Fundamentalism and the resurgence of religion." *Numen* 47.3 (2000): 266–287.
26 Samuels, Robert. "Catharsis: The politics of enjoyment." In Robert Samuels, *Žižek and the rhetorical unconscious: Global politics, philosophy, and subjectivity*. Springer, 2020: 7–31.

27 Forrester, John. "Lacan's debt to Freud: how the Ratman paid off his debt." In Todd Dufresne (ed.), *Returns of the French Freud: Freud, Lacan, and beyond.* Routledge, 2013: 67–89.
28 Huaco, George A. "Ideology and general theory: The case of sociological functionalism." *Comparative Studies in Society and History* 28.1 (1986): 34–54.
29 Allcorn, Seth. "Binaries: Psychodynamic insights in a world view split apart." *The Journal of Psychohistory* 50.1 (2022): 2–15.
30 Samuels, Robert, and Robert Samuels. "Behavioral economics: Nudge and technocratic liberalism." In Robert Samuels, *Psychoanalyzing the politics of the new brain sciences.* Springer, 2017: 59–83.
31 Rose, Steven, Richard Charles Lewontin, and Leon Kamin. "Not in our genes: Biology, ideology and human nature." *The Wilson Quarterly* 152 (1984).
32 Dijk, Teun A. van. "Discourse, opinions and ideologies." *Current Issues in Language & Society* 2.2 (1995): 115–145.
33 Weissenbacher, Alan. "Sally Satel and Scott Lilienfeld, *Brainwashed: The Seductive Appeal of Mindless Neuroscience.*" *Theology & Science* 12.1 (2014): 119–121.
34 Samuels, Robert. "The metaphorical misunderstanding AI and ourselves." In Robert Samuels, *The global solution to AI: Risks, rhetoric, ideology, and psychoanalysis.* Palgrave Macmillan, 2025: 27–48.
35 Samuels, Robert. *Psychoanalyzing the politics of the new brain sciences.* Springer, 2017.
36 Larregue, Julien, and Sylvain Lavau. "Evolutionary psychology and the naturalization of gender inequalities." *Science & Technology Studies* 38.1 (2025): 61–74.
37 Jackson, Stevi, and Amanda Rees. "The appalling appeal of nature: The popular influence of evolutionary psychology as a problem for sociology." *Sociology* 41.5 (2007): 917–930.
38 Samuels, Robert. "Neuro-psychoanalysis and the representation of humans as biological machines." In Robert Samuels, *The global solution to AI: Risks, rhetoric, ideology, and psychoanalysis.* Palgrave Macmillan, 2025: 77–97.
39 Samuels, Robert. "The backlash politics of evolutionary psychology: Steven Pinker's blank slate." In Robert Samuels, *Psychoanalyzing the politics of the new brain sciences.* Springer, 2017: 35–58.
40 Daempfle, Peter A. *Good science, bad science, pseudoscience, and just plain bunk: How to tell the difference.* Rowman & Littlefield Publishers, 2012.
41 Galston, William A. "Two concepts of liberalism." *Ethics* 105.3 (1995): 516–534.
42 Samuels, Robert. *Culture wars, universities, and the political unconscious.* Palgrave Macmillan, 2024.
43 Kenny, Anthony. "Myths of the mind and myths of the brain." *Philosophical Inquiries* 1.1 (2013): 63–72.
44 Cavell, Marcia. "Dividing the self." In Gerhard Preyer, Frank Siebelt, and Alexander Ulfig (eds.), *Language, mind and epistemology: On Donald Davidson's philosophy.* Springer, 1994: 299–311.
45 Samuels, Robert. *The psychoanalytic understanding of consciousness, free will, language, and reason: What makes us human?* Routledge, 2023.
46 Tougaw, Jason. "Before neuromania." In Jason Tougaw, *The elusive brain: Literary experiments in the age of neuroscience.* Yale University Press, 2018: 39.
47 Freud, Sigmund. *Group psychology and the analysis of the ego.* Hogarth Press, 1949.
48 Modell, Arnold H. "The evolutionary significance of the primary process—The Freudian concept and its revision." *Psychoanalytic Inquiry* 34.8 (2014): 810–816.
49 Foster, Mary LeCron. "Analogy, language, and the symbolic process." In Mary Lecron Foster and Lucy Jayne Botscharow (eds.), *The life of symbols.* Routledge, 2019: 81–94.

50 Clift, Wallace, and Jean Dalby Clift. "Symbols of transformation in dreams." In David A. Leeming (ed.), *Encyclopedia of psychology and religion*. Springer, 2020: 2319–2322.
51 De Masi, Franco, et al. "Hallucinations in the psychotic state: Psychoanalysis and the neurosciences compared." *The International Journal of Psychoanalysis* 96.2 (2015): 293–318.
52 Federn, Paul. "Ego feeling in dreams." *The Psychoanalytic Review (1913–1957)* 26 (1939): 438.
53 Spiegel, Herbert. "Hypnosis and transference: A theoretical formulation." *AMA Archives of General Psychiatry* 1.6 (1959): 634–639.
54 Freud, Sigmund. *Moses and monotheism*. Sanzani Edizioni, 2023.
55 Bernheim, B. Douglas, and Christine Exley. Understanding conformity: An experimental investigation. NOM Unit Working Paper 16-070, Harvard Business School, 2015.
56 Reed, Gail S. "The transference neurosis in Freud's writings." *Journal of the American Psychoanalytic Association* 38.2 (1990): 423–450.
57 Freud, Sigmund. "The dynamics of transference." In James Strachey (ed.), The standard edition of the complete psychological works of Sigmund Freud. Vol. 12. Hogarth Press, 1953–1974: 108.
58 O'Gieblyn, Meghan. *God, human, animal, machine: Technology, metaphor, and the search for meaning*. Vintage, 2022.
59 Samuels, Robert. "The metaphorical misunderstanding: AI and ourselves." In Robert Samuels, *The global solution to AI: Risks, rhetoric, ideology, and psychoanalysis*. Palgrave Macmillan, 2025: 27–48.
60 Samuels, Robert. "The metaphorical misunderstanding: AI and ourselves." In Robert Samuels, *The global solution to AI: Risks, rhetoric, ideology, and psychoanalysis*. Palgrave Macmillan, 2025: 27–48.
61 Samuels, Richard. "Science and human nature." *Royal Institute of Philosophy Supplements* 70 (2012): 1–28.
62 Samuels, Robert. *The psychoanalytic understanding of consciousness, free will, language, and reason: What makes us human?*. Routledge, 2023.
63 Samuels, Robert, and Robert Samuels. "Damasio's error: The politics of biological determinism after Freud." *Psychoanalyzing the politics of the new brain sciences* (2017): 9–33.
64 Pagden, Anthony. *The Enlightenment: and why it still matters*. Oxford University Press, 2013.
65 Descartes, René. *A discourse on method*. J. M. Dent & Sons, 1929.
66 Samuels, Robert. "Science and the reality principle." In Robert Samuels, *Freud for the twenty-first century: The science of everyday life* (2019): 5–16.
67 Chalmers, David. "The hard problem of consciousness." In Susan Schneider and Max Velmans (eds.), *The Blackwell companion to consciousness*. Blackwell, 2017: 32–42.
68 Derksen, Anthony A. "The seven sins of pseudo-science." *Journal for General Philosophy of Science* 24 (1993): 17–42.
69 Yablo, Stephen. "The real distinction between mind and body." *Canadian Journal of Philosophy supplementary volume* 16 (1990): 149–201.
70 Hurry, Anne, Jack Novick, and Kerry Kelly Novick. "Freud's concept of projection." *Journal of Child Psychotherapy* 4.2 (1976): 75–88.
71 Knight, Robert P. "Introjection, projection and identification." *The Psychoanalytic Quarterly* 9.3 (1940): 334–341.

Chapter 5

Aristotle's *Rhetoric* and the Center-Right Justification for Social Hierarchy and Inequality

Aristotle's *Rhetoric* provides a deep insight into how social hierarchies and inequalities are often justified and rationalized through the use of metaphorical thinking and a center-Right ideology.[1] Moreover, as Nietzsche insists, the social and personal traits that Aristotle idealizes also happen to be the traits that represent Aristotle's own idealized self.[2] Thus, we can understand his discourse as being shaped by a combination of traditionalism and narcissism as he desires to show why it is necessary and natural for a social hierarchy that he profits from to exist. Moreover, his use of nature to define culture and psychology anticipates the ways the brain sciences now often seek to comprehend ideology today. What we discover by examining Aristotle's words is that he unknowingly articulates the psychological foundations of wealthy-white-male privilege and center-Right ideology.

The Discourse of the Master

To understand how Aristotle views his own cultural order, we can look at an important passage from his *Politics*:[3]

> for the soul rules the body with a despotical rule, whereas the intellect rules the appetites with a constitutional and royal rule. And it is clear that the rule of the soul over the body, and of the mind and the rational element over the passionate, is natural and expedient; whereas the equality of the two or the rule of the inferior is always hurtful. The same holds good of animals in relation to men; for tame animals have a better nature than wild, and all tame animals are better off when they are ruled by man; for then they are preserved. Again, the male is by nature superior, and the female inferior; and the one rules, and the other is ruled; this principle, of necessity, extends to all mankind … the lower sort are by nature slaves, and it is better for them as for all inferiors that they should be under the rule of a master.
>
> (Aristotle, *Politics*, book 1, part V)

DOI: 10.4324/9781003773948-5

This passage offers us great insight into Aristotle's prejudices and shows how these stereotypes still structure much of our lives today and the world around us.[4] In many ways, Aristotle is exposing the foundations of center-Right ideology, which is based on naturalizing his culture's particular social hierarchies: men are privileged over women, masters over slaves, reason over emotion, and humans over animals.[5] It is important to stress that for most of human history, these hierarchies have dominated our world and that the effort to treat these social relations as natural is one of the central rhetorical strategies of the center-Right.[6] After all, if something is natural, then it cannot be changed because it has been predetermined by some higher power or natural order.[7]

From a modern liberal perspective, we know that social hierarchies are not natural, and they can be transformed, yet people still often try to persuade others to accept these prejudices by claiming that they are based on some type of natural or divine order.[8] Since Aristotle wants to argue that the character of the speaker plays an important role in rhetoric, and as we shall see, this character is defined in relation to the social hierarchy, it is vital to both understand and critique the dominant cultural order shaping authority and character (ethos).[9] Moreover, how Aristotle justifies slavery and patriarchy reveals the ways political ideologies are constructed through the manipulation of language.[10]

On the most basic level, Aristotle defines his own character as good and the opposite of his self-definition as bad.[11] Since he is a free human male using his intellect to reason, he sees his character as superior to disempowered females and slaves who are defined by their association with emotion, the body, and animal instincts.[12] Language plays the key role here by using the logic of opposition to produce a set of binary differences.[13] In turn, these oppositions create a set of symbolic analogies and associations: just as men are represented as being superior to women, masters are superior to slaves, and reason is superior to emotion.[14] Moreover, women become associated with the traits of the body, animals, slaves, and emotions.[15]

Through the use of oppositions, analogies, and associations, Aristotle reveals the rhetorical foundations of his social order.[16] Furthermore, we see how there is a self-justifying rationalization driving his language use since he is not only defining what he sees to be the structure of his culture, but he is also saying that it is natural and expedient for people like himself to have power, authority, and ultimately, privilege.[17] However, there is a logical contradiction in his argument since he is using nature both to indicate what determines each relation and to define what is inferior to culture; from his perspective, it is natural for humans to dominate animals because humans have intellect, and animals are shaped by natural instincts.[18]

Of course, Aristotle does not discuss his contradictory usage of nature, yet we can read this contradiction as pointing to the ways people seek to prove their arguments and worldviews by confusing what is natural with what is cultural.[19] Since nature is seen as universal and inevitable, when you claim that some social relation is natural, you shut down any possibility of change as you justify the social status quo.[20] This strategy of naturalizing social constructions still functions today even though it goes against the modern scientific and secular perspective, and so it is productive to understand the logic of center-Right ideology and naturalization. Moreover, we not only see how linguistic oppositions, analogies, and associations structure philosophical arguments, but we also encounter how sexism and racism can reinforce each other and how they often rely on implicit cultural connections that become naturalized over time.[21]

Modern Reason and Aristotle

One of the challenges facing the contemporary reader of Aristotle is that some of his arguments fit in well with modern liberal scientific and democratic values, yet others are in direct conflict, and thus we have to find ways to separate the two.[22] We can begin to address this problem of historical and cultural relativism by looking at the following passage on the role of rhetoric in legal proceedings:

> The arousing of prejudice, pity, anger, and similar emotions has nothing to do with the essential facts, but is merely a personal appeal to the man who is judging the case. Consequently if the rules for trials which are now laid down in some states—especially in well-governed states—were applied everywhere, such people would have nothing to say. All men, no doubt, think that the laws should prescribe such rules, but some, as in the court of Areopagus, give practical effect to their thoughts and forbid talk about non-essentials. This is sound law and custom. It is not right to pervert the judge by moving him to anger or envy or pity—one might as well warp a carpenter's rule before using it. Again, a litigant has clearly nothing to do but to show that the alleged fact is so or is not so, that it has or has not happened.
>
> (*R*: 13)

On one level, this argument for the appeal to reason (logos) and not emotion (pathos) in legal cases appears to be very modern since a key aspect of democratic law since the Enlightenment is the idea that the judge needs to apply reason in an impartial way based purely on the evidence and not on feelings of pity or prejudice.[23] However, we know that for Aristotle, only wealthy, free men with property were seen to have reason, and so we need to understand that his use of reason is defined by his social hierarchy and privilege.[24]

For many Leftist postmodern thinkers, this call to use neutral reason (logos) always hides a vested class interest, and since it was white male

Europeans who came up with the idea of modern reason, this ideology can only result in prejudice and discrimination.[25] Yet, we must consider objectivity, reason, and impartiality as impossible but necessary liberal ideals that shape our modern global democratic and scientific institutions. In fact, the critique of modern reason uses reason to make its argument, and thus when we criticize a system for not being fair and just, we are judging the system against the modern ideals of reason and equality.[26] We have to therefore learn to examine critically our modern institutions without rejecting them completely. In fact, Aristotle's rhetoric is so fruitful because it exposes this conflicted relationship between traditional hierarchy and modern equality.[27]

Although Aristotle is limited by his belief that his social hierarchy is the product of natural order, he is still able to point to the key role of logos as reason in modern democratic law:

> The weightiest reason of all is that the decision of the lawgiver is not particular but prospective and general, whereas members of the assembly and the jury find it their duty to decide on definite cases brought before them. They will often have allowed themselves to be so much influenced by feelings of friendship or hatred or self-interest that they lose any clear vision of the truth and have their judgement obscured by considerations of personal pleasure or pain.
>
> (*R*: 14)

Aristotle makes several important points here concerning the role of logos (reason) in democratic law.[28] The first idea is that law has to be general and not personal even though people have a hard time thinking beyond their own prejudices and self-interests. In fact, we have seen that Aristotle himself has a self-interested, prejudicial view of the world, and yet he also points to a way out of this traditional ideology.[29] By privileging facts and reason over feelings and prejudice, he endorses the liberal democratic ideal that the law should be impersonal and universal; from this perspective, empathy and pity are not the key to modern democratic law and liberal ideology since these feelings can often be biased and self-interested.[30]

While many on the center-Left may believe that empathy is the driving force behind equality, Aristotle reveals why modern universal democratic law has to suspend the pathos of sympathy and emotional connection in order to use logos in a neutral way.[31] Although his argument does not mean that emotion (pathos) does not play a vital role in communication and politics, it does affirm that we need to learn how to separate these rhetorical modes and ideologies in order to determine in which contexts they are the most appropriate.[32] In fact, all forms of communication utilize pathos, logos, and ethos to a certain extent because when we communicate, our audience has to trust our character (ethos), and we have to believe that the audience will be able to use reason (logos) to understand what we are saying.[33] Furthermore, no one will listen to us if they do not have some interest in what we are discussing, and this interest is always based on emotions (pathos) and desire. The issue then is what mode of rhetoric is given priority in each particular context (kairos).[34]

Truth and Nature

Like many contemporary neuroscientists and evolutionary psychologists, underlying Aristotle's discourse is a belief in natural order:

> Rhetoric is useful because things that are true and things that are just have a natural tendency to prevail over their opposites, so that if the decisions of judges are not what they ought to be, the defeat must be due to the speakers themselves, and they must be blamed accordingly.
>
> (*R*: 15)

Since Aristotle believes that there is a natural law and order, he thinks that true things will prevail over untrue things.[35] While this notion of natural law may seem absurd to many contemporary readers, it actually is at the foundation of many current authoritarian and traditional legal theories and practices.[36] Since originalists want to believe that there is a discoverable natural order to the legal system, they believe they can interpret texts like the U.S. constitution without taking into account any contexts.[37] This method of interpretation is in part derived from the way certain religions read texts on a supposedly literal level. Due to the need to eliminate the human interference between God and the word, all contexts have to be removed, and yet secular liberals know this to be an impossibility.[38]

Although it is unclear what causes natural law for Aristotle, it has the same logic as a divine order.[39] Once again, at the heart of this center-Right discourse, there is often a belief in natural order: "things that are true and things that are better are, by their nature, practically always easier to prove and easier to believe in" (*R*: 16). This idea that true things are easier to prove and accept clearly contradicts our lived experience, and so it can only be the result of Aristotle's investment in the ideology of natural order.[40] While he wants to believe that the best things are true, and the truth is always best, we know that rhetoric is often used to persuade people to believe in falsehoods.[41]

Aristotle's Communication Model

The continued influence of Aristotle's thought can be seen in his definition of the basic structure of communication:

> Of the modes of persuasion furnished by the spoken word there are three kinds. The first kind depends on the personal character of the speaker; the or apparent proof, provided by the words of the speech itself.

> Persuasion is achieved by the speaker's personal character when the speech is so spoken as to make us think him credible. We believe good men more fully and more readily than others: this is true generally whatever the question is, and absolutely true where exact certainty is impossible and opinions are divided.
>
> (*R*: 17)

For Aristotle, the ethos of a speaker is defined by character, which itself has to be understood in relation to a particular social hierarchy.[42] However, in contemporary society, this hierarchy is contested, and so we need to think about the ways credibility is established outside of an aristocratic order. For instance, academic writers often determine the credibility of a source based on the institutional status of the writer; a professor from Harvard is supposed to have credibility not because of his character but because of the processes related to peer-reviewed publications.[43] From the position of modern liberal ideology, one is not born into a position of authority; rather, credibility has to be established through the rigors of scientific methodology and peer review.[44]

In the case of Aristotle's understanding of ethos based on the perceived character of the speaker, credibility is derived in relation to the pre-established social hierarchy:

> It is not true, as some writers assume in their treatises on rhetoric, that the personal goodness revealed by the speaker contributes nothing to his power of persuasion; on the contrary, his character may almost be called the most effective means of persuasion he possesses. Secondly, persuasion may come through the hearers, when the speech stirs their emotions. Our judgements when we are pleased and friendly are not the same as when we are pained and hostile.
>
> (*R*: 17)

From Aristotle's privileged perspective, the speaker's discourse is framed by the audience's understanding of the personal goodness of the orator.[45] Even when pathos, in the form of an emotional appeal, is utilized, this mode of rhetoric relies on the perceived ethos of the speaker; thus, for Aristotle, ethos determines how the other modes of rhetoric will be received by the audience.

Importantly, the three main modes of rhetoric—ethos, logos, and pathos—are first presented as connected forms of persuasion:

> The man who is to be in command of them must, it is clear, be able (1) to reason logically, (2) to understand human character and goodness in their various forms, and (3) to understand the emotions—that is, to name them and describe them, to know their causes and the way in which they are excited.
>
> (*R*: 17)

These appeals to reason (logos), character (ethos), and emotion (pathos) still serve as the basic way we understand rhetoric and ideology today.[46] From this perspective, each belief system is derived from a particular relational desire encoded in a specific mode of appeal and persuasion.[47] For instance, we can consider ethos as the foundation of the authoritarian desire for salvation mixed with the traditional social order, while logos points to the liberal democratic call for truth and universality. Moreover, appeals based on emotion (pathos) play a key role in Leftist and center-Left ideologies because the goal is to make people care about the suffering of oppressed individuals or groups.[48] Here we see that distinct ideologies present extreme forms of rhetorical appeals.

The Science of Reason

Although Aristotle never examines the relative and arbitrary nature of the social values determined by his own traditional culture, he does seek to establish a universal science of language and communication:

> But none of the arts theorize about individual cases. Medicine, for instance, does not theorize about what will help to cure Socrates or Callias, but only about what will help to cure any or all of a given class of patients: this alone is its business: individual cases are so infinitely various that no systematic knowledge of them is possible.
>
> (*R*: 18–19)

Instead of seeing universality as a necessary but impossible ideal for science, Aristotle seeks to base his rhetoric on a generalized discourse that goes beyond any particular instances.[49]

As part of his desire to establish a science of communication, Aristotle needs to determine the roles played by language in representing truth to others, and one of the main ways that he attempts to establish the transparency of language is by developing his concept of infallible signs:

> By infallible signs I mean those on which syllogisms proper may be based: and this shows us why this kind of Sign is called "complete proof": when people think that what they have said cannot be refuted, they then think that they are bringing forward a "complete proof," meaning that the matter has now been demonstrated and completed.
>
> (*R*: 20)

We see here how his entire theory is based on the ideal of clear, rational communication, and so even if people misunderstand each other or signs have multiple significations, it is necessary to posit an ideal of complete and transparent communication:

> Suppose it were said, "The fact that Socrates was wise and just is a sign that the wise are just." Here we certainly have a Sign; but even though the proposition be true, the argument is refutable, since it does not form a syllogism. Suppose, on the other hand, it were said, "The fact that he has a fever is a sign that he is ill," or, "The fact that she is giving milk is a sign that she has lately borne a child." Here we have the infallible kind of Sign, the only kind that constitutes a complete proof, since it is the only kind that, if the particular statement is true, is irrefutable.
>
> (*R*: 20)

While psychoanalysis has discovered that it is possible for people to have a fever when they are not ill and for women to produce milk when they are not pregnant, Aristotle has to posit the possibility of infallible signs in order to base his science on received knowledge and not empirical testing.[50] Thus, unlike modern science, center-Right ideology relies on accepted generalizations in order to make seemingly rational claims.

One reason why Aristotle's theories of rhetoric and communication are insightful is that they ground language in social relationships structured by what he calls the three categories of speech:

> Rhetoric falls into three divisions, determined by the three classes of listeners to speeches. For of the three elements in speech-making—speaker, subject, and person addressed—it is the last one, the hearer, that determines the speech's end and object. The hearer must be either a judge, with a decision to make about things past or future, or an observer. A member of the assembly decides about future events, a juryman about past events: while those who merely decide on the orator's skill are observers. From this it follows that there are three divisions of oratory—(1) political, (2) forensic, and (3) the ceremonial oratory of display.
>
> (*R*: 22)

Aristotle's triadic logic begins by separating the speaker from the content and the audience. From his perspective, the audience determines the meaning of the speech act, and this role of the audience is shaped by the context, which relates to the situation being one of politics, law, or ceremony.[51] Moreover, the political audience is seen as dealing with the future, while the legal judge relates to past events, and the ceremonial audience to the present oration. The temporality of the speech act thus serves to contextualize each aspect of rhetoric, and so we can consider the context as a fourth determining factor along with the speaker, the content, and the audience.[52] As a way of addressing the underlying relational desires that shape specific ideologies, Aristotle's theory points to the need to think of belief systems as structuring the relations among speakers, audiences, and social contexts.

The Pursuit of Happiness

Driving Aristotle's theory of rhetoric is his seemingly libertarian belief that humans are driven by their pursuit of happiness:

> It may be said that every individual man and all men in common aim at a certain end which determines what they choose and what they avoid. This end, to sum it up briefly, is happiness and its constituents. Let us, then, by way of illustration only, ascertain what is in general the nature of happiness, and what are the elements of its constituent parts. For all advice to do things or not to do them is concerned with happiness and with the things that make for or against it; whatever creates or increases happiness or some part of happiness, we ought to do; whatever destroys or hampers happiness, or gives rise to its opposite, we ought not to do.
>
> (*R*: 26–27)

Aristotle here appears to anticipate Freud's notion that the pleasure principle is the fundamental drive shaping human subjectivity and that pleasure itself is defined by the desire to escape tension, anxiety, and displeasure.[53]

Aristotle's endorsement of a libertarian ideology is most clear when he defines the role of happiness in politics, culture, and psychology:

> We may define happiness as prosperity combined with virtue; or as independence of life; or as the secure enjoyment of the maximum of pleasure; or as a good condition of property and body, together with the power of guarding one's property and body and making use of them.
>
> (*R*: 27)

This passage sounds eerily like the rhetoric we hear from the mouths of Right-wing politicians and activists: From this perspective, humans are driven by the desire for life, liberty, and pleasure.[54] However, for Aristotle, this libertarian ideology is framed by an underlying investment in a natural social order.

Just as Aristotle defines the master as the one who is good because he is a free male with power and social position, he equates happiness with the privileges of the master patriarch.[55] After all, it is only the wealthy, secure, prosperous, property-owning, free male who is seen as representing the one whose happiness defines his pursuits.[56] Although we may find this sexist and classist perspective oppressive, it does point to how human civilization has been shaped by the ability of a powerful minority of mostly men to determine what is seen as good and pleasurable.[57]

Of course, Aristotle never seems to realize that his definition of happiness and good character (ethos) relies on simply representing his own attributes as ideal:

> From this definition of happiness it follows that its constituent parts are:—good birth, plenty of friends, good friends, wealth, good children, plenty of children, a happy old age, also such bodily excellences as health, beauty, strength, large stature, athletic powers, together with fame, honour, good luck, and virtue. A man cannot fail to be completely independent if he possesses these internal and these external goods; for besides these there are no others to have. (Goods of the soul and of the body are internal. Good birth, friends, money, and honour are external.) Further, we think that he should possess resources and luck, in order to make his life really secure.
>
> (*R*: 27)

The ethos of the speaker is thus defined by the pursuit of happiness, which itself is associated with a good birth, wealth, health, fame, honor, and security.[58] From this elitist, aristocratic perspective, everything good and positive is the result of inherited wealth and social position.[59] Once again, while we may find this ideology to be outmoded and odious, it still shapes our world because so much of wealth is still the direct or indirect result of inheritance.[60]

It is also vital to see that Aristotle's conception of pleasure and happiness connects his theory of communication to his theory of aesthetics:

> Pleasure, again, must be a good thing, since it is the nature of all animals to aim at it. Consequently both pleasant and beautiful things must be good things, since the former are productive of pleasure, while of the beautiful things some are pleasant and some desirable in and for themselves.
>
> (*R*: 30–31)

Since all animals are driven by the pursuit of pleasure, and beautiful things produce pleasure, Aristotle posits that the effective use of language must be beautiful and pleasurable.[61] However, as we have seen, pleasure and beauty are themselves determined by a self-reinforcing social hierarchy centered on cultural stereotypes, prejudices, and discriminations.[62]

From a modern perspective, we know that beauty and pleasure are relative to a particular culture and time period, so what Aristotle considers to be natural and universal must be seen as un-natural and historical.[63] Yet, the social hierarchies he describes still affect our social worlds on a daily basis because they represent many of the default settings of our cultural attitudes. Therefore, as the world becomes less defined by the old traditional ideology, there are still many resistances to these changes as people try to maintain the original system of social hierarchies.[64]

In terms of rhetoric and ideology, it is important to realize how the definition of ethos as the authority of the speaker or writer is shaped by internalized social definitions of authority and cultural value.[65] Furthermore,

Aristotle points to the ways rhetoric seeks to produce happiness by appearing to be beautiful and pleasurable, but pleasure and beauty themselves must be seen as being relative to a particular culture, history, and context. In fact, I will argue below that besides the three rhetorical appeals of ethos, logos, and pathos, we should also consider catharsis as the pleasure produced through art and other cultural productions.[66] Whereas Aristotle does not make this connection in his book on rhetoric, he does define catharsis in his *Poetics* as the audience's release of feelings of pity and fear while watching a play.[67] As a form of happiness and pleasure, catharsis relies on releasing the individual from any pent up feelings or pathos.[68]

Aristotle's Traditional Ideology Reconsidered

The paradox of Aristotle's view of the world is that he sees everything as determined by social class, and yet, he still thinks that these class distinctions are natural and inevitable.[69] In relation to rhetoric, he argues that people are only concerned about maintaining the current social order:

> For all men are persuaded by considerations of their interest, and their interest lies in the maintenance of the established order. Further, it rests with the supreme authority to give authoritative decisions, and this varies with each form of government.
>
> (*R*: 38–39)

On one level, traditional ideology is driven by this desire for social order; however, on another level, it opens up the door for an authoritarian ideology where one submits to the idealized supreme authority.[70]

Once again, the reason why Aristotle is able to equate interest, happiness, and the status quo is that he defines pleasure as conforming to a natural state:

> We may lay it down that Pleasure is a movement, a movement by which the soul as a whole is consciously brought into its normal state of being; and that Pain is the opposite. If this is what pleasure is, it is clear that the pleasant is what tends to produce this condition, while that which tends to destroy it, or to cause the soul to be brought into the opposite state, is painful. It must therefore be pleasant as a rule to move towards a natural state of being, particularly when a natural process has achieved the complete recovery of that natural state. Habits also are pleasant; for as soon as a thing has become habitual, it is virtually natural; habit is a thing not unlike nature; what happens often is akin to what happens always, natural events happening always, habitual events often. Again, that is pleasant which is not forced on us; for force is unnatural, and that is why what is compulsory is painful.
>
> (*R*: 47–48)

In the passage above, we see how important Aristotle's rhetorical use of "nature" is to his whole philosophy and worldview.[71] To rationalize his own power and privilege, he constantly returns to the notion that what he values and what his society privileges is the result of a natural order, and therefore it is universal and unchangeable. By defining his own attributes as ideal, he tries to persuade his audience that the system granting him social power and authority is simply natural and inevitable.[72] To counter this rhetoric, we have to call into question this use of nature as an ideological rationalization of an oppressive social hierarchy. While Aristotle insists that what is natural is what occurs without force, we know that his social hierarchy is enforced through violence and the threat of harm.[73]

It is important to stress how much of Aristotle's view of rhetoric is shaped by his particular social position. As a wealthy white male who has the time and resources to contemplate the world in a safe and secure way, he defines pleasure by the absence of effort and strain:

> So all acts of concentration, strong effort, and strain are necessarily painful; they all involve compulsion and force, unless we are accustomed to them, in which case it is custom that makes them pleasant. The opposites to these are pleasant; and hence ease, freedom from toil, relaxation, amusement, rest, and sleep belong to the class of pleasant things; for these are all free from any element of compulsion. Everything, too, is pleasant for which we have the desire within us, since desire is the craving for pleasure.
>
> (*R*: 48)

While for Freud, the pleasure principle is defined by the universal desire to avoid or release all conflict and tension, for Aristotle, this type of pleasure is related to the way his class has the ability to be free from toil and any type of social compulsion.[74] It is therefore necessary to emphasize how his ideology is shaped by a class perspective, which idealizes his attributes and devalues the opposing traits of people without the same social power and resources.

As a center-Right thinker, Aristotle's sense of reason (*logos*) has to be understood through his constant naturalization of social hierarchies and class positions. For instance, when he attempts to separate reason from unreason, he relies on his implicit equating of natural order and cultural order:

> Of the desires some are irrational, some associated with reason. By irrational I mean those which do not arise from any opinion held by the mind. Of this kind are those known as "natural"; for instance, those originating in the body, such as the desire for nourishment, namely hunger and thirst, and a separate kind of desire answering to each kind of nourishment; and the desires connected with taste and sex and sensations of touch in general; and those of smell, hearing, and vision.

> Rational desires are those which we are induced to have; there are many things we desire to see or get because we have been told of them and induced to believe them good.
>
> (*R*: 48)

From this traditional perspective, reason (logos) is associated with mental opinions derived from the social definition of goodness.[75] In other words, center-Right reason is shaped by prejudice and self-interest, and in this way, it contrasts with the modern liberal notion that reason should be universal, impersonal, and neutral.

Not only does Aristotle understand reason through his social class position, but his sense of emotion (pathos) is also shaped by social hierarchy: "for no one grows angry with a person on whom there is no prospect of taking vengeance, and we feel comparatively little anger, or none at all, with those who are much our superiors in power" (*R*: 49). Aristotle reveals here why we need to think of emotions as mediated by social perceptions instead of being purely natural biological reactions.[76] In fact, although we often experience emotions as being automatic responses, Aristotle helps us to think about pathos from a cultural and psychological perspective. Writing 2000 years before Freud, his understanding of emotion points to the roles played by imagination and non-conscious processes in shaping our subjective experiences:

> Some pleasant feeling is associated with most of our appetites; we are enjoying either the memory of a past pleasure or the expectation of a future one, just as persons down with fever, during their attacks of thirst, enjoy remembering the drinks they have had and looking forward to having more. So also a lover enjoys talking or writing about his loved one, or doing any little thing connected with him; all these things recall him to memory and make him actually present to the eye of imagination.
>
> (*R*: 49)

It is, then, the power of human memory to recall symbolic associations connected to past experiences that enables imagination and subjectivity.[77] For Freud, this power of imagination defines conscious thought as the ability to perceive memories of past events, and it is this concept of the primary processes that shapes the irrational foundation of emotions.[78] Moreover, since emotions are structured by social and psychological symbolic networks, they utilize natural responses in an unnatural way.

Narcissism and Social Status

Due to the fact that Aristotle believes that his view of the world is natural and universal, he does not recognize the importance of how his own social position shapes the ways he sees the world and himself. In fact, when he does discuss the social influence of individual psychology, he tends to adopt a narcissistic view:

> it is pleasant to be loved, for this too makes a man see himself as the possessor of goodness, a thing that every being that has a feeling for it desires to possess: to be loved means to be valued for one's own personal qualities. To be admired is also pleasant, simply because of the honour implied. Flattery and flatterers are pleasant: the flatterer is a man who, you believe, admires and likes you. To do the same thing often is pleasant, since, as we saw, anything habitual is pleasant.
>
> (*R*: 50)

This passage displays the connections Aristotle makes among narcissism, the pleasure principle, and ethos.[79] Since it is pleasant to be admired, one's social character is reinforced by the way social status is recognized by others.[80] It is thus not good enough for the powerful male authority to see himself as good; he also has to have others recognize his goodness, and this recognition of the social hierarchy is seen as producing pleasure because it is habitual. Here we find the essence of narcissism and center-Right ideology: Since people desire to be admired for their goodness, they have to conform to what their society considered to be ideal.[81]

Like everything else in Aristotle's rhetoric, his sense of art is also defined by a focus on a class-based experience of pleasure through imitation:

> Again, since learning and wondering are pleasant, it follows that such things as acts of imitation must be pleasant—for instance, painting, sculpture, poetry—and every product of skilful imitation; this latter, even if the object imitated is not itself pleasant; for it is not the object itself which here gives delight; the spectator draws inferences ("That is a so-and-so") and thus learns something fresh.
>
> (*R*: 50)

Aristotle posits here that learning and artistic imitation are pleasurable because they both provide the audience with a new way of seeing the world.[82] Yet, he has previously argued that what is habitual is by nature pleasant, and so it is hard to understand how new knowledge can also be considered to be a source of pleasure. The way he gets around this conflict is by returning to his theory of nature: "And since what is natural is pleasant, and things akin to each other seem natural to each other, therefore all kindred and similar things are usually pleasant to each other" (*R*: 51). So even if imitation or learning teaches us something new, what we find pleasant is the discovery of the natural connection between specific things.[83] From his center-Right perspective, we are told that traditional art, culture, and education are ideal because they are all based on the pleasure of finding natural connections between similar things. Tradition, custom, fate, and natural order therefore reinforce each other through Aristotle's theory of pleasure, but as we saw above, this endorsement of traditional ideology is itself framed by a desire for self-idealization, which underlies center-Right ideology.[84] On the most basic level, the naturalization of privilege and the idealization of the ego allow for one to escape and feelings of guilt and shame related to profiting from an unequal society.

One reason why it so important to understand Aristotle's center-Right ideology is that this philosopher helps us to comprehend how current pundits, politicians, and philosophers provide ideological cover for social inequality and hierarchy. In fact, I argue that much of Western philosophy and psychology is based on an attempt to naturalize and justify the privileges of wealthy white males. As we currently find in many different popular podcasts and YouTube videos, the destructive effects of libertarian and authoritarian ideologies are hidden by center-Right apologists who use their own privilege to idealize economic and social inequality. As a new form of social Darwinism, this aristocratic class pretends to be liberal as it enables the Right-wing counter-revolution.

In fact, not only does Aristotle insist that similar people find pleasure in recognizing their shared attributes: He also theorizes that people love themselves because they are more like themselves than they are like other people:

> since every man is himself more like and akin to himself than any one else is, it follows that all of us must be more or less fond of ourselves. For all this resemblance and kinship is present particularly in the relation of an individual to himself. And because we are all fond of ourselves, it follows that what is our own is pleasant to all of us, as for instance our own deeds and words. That is why we are usually fond of our flatterers, [our lovers,] and honour; also of our children, for our children are our own work.
>
> (*R*: 51)

Since pleasure is defined by the recognition of natural sameness or similarity, we love ourselves and the people who are most like us.[85] Of course, we know that some people do not love themselves, and ethnocentrism, prejudice, and stereotypes are often derived from our focus on privileging our own traits as superior to others, yet from Aristotle's center-Right view, social hierarchy and the idealization of the ego are the same thing: we love's others who remind us of ourselves and who recognize our exalted place within the social hierarchy.[86] What happens with modernity and its liberal ideology is that the social hierarchy will be replaced by the claim for equality as the public and private realms become separated; modernity thus threatens social narcissism because self-worth becomes dissociated from the social hierarchy and natural order.[87]

Ultimately, Aristotle's narcissistic view of his social hierarchy is based on naturalizing his privilege and justifying the distribution of power within his culture:

> And since power over others is very pleasant, it is pleasant to be thought wise, for practical wisdom secures us power over others. (Scientific wisdom is also pleasant, because it is the knowledge of many wonderful things.) Again, since most of us are ambitious, it must be pleasant to disparage our neighbours as well as to have power over them.
>
> (*R*: 51)

For a contemporary reader, this blatant celebration of social power and the disparagement of the disempowered may appear off-putting, yet it is important to think about how Aristotle is exposing underlying aspects of past and present social hierarchies and privilege.[88]On the one hand, we want to describe how universal claims are often shaped by covert self-interest, but on the other hand, we also need to see how authority as ethos functions in all acts of communication.

Pragmatic Idealism

One of the underlying claims of my understanding of rhetoric and ideology is that we communicate by assuming a series of necessary but impossible ideals.[89] Thus, we assume that we can be understood and that our audience will make a good faith effort to use reason to process what we say. We also assume that our words represent reality and that our language is a transparent medium, which allows our internal thoughts to be circulated in an external form without distortion. Of course, philosophers and psychologists have shown how all of these assumptions are prone to error, yet I would argue that in order to critique this theory of pragmatic idealism, one has to act like a pragmatic idealist.[90] In other words, there is no way to reject reason without using reason, and there is no reason to communicate at all, if you do not believe that your words can be understood, and these symbols relate to a shared reality.

In terms of rhetoric and ideology, we cannot escape assuming that there is an author, a content, a context, and an audience for each act of persuasion.[91] We also have to affirm that the author relates to authority and ethos as defined by a particular social hierarchy, and the audience and the speaker will use logos as reason in order to understand each other. Moreover, pathos is always involved since people will only pay attention to a persuasive communication if they are interested in the subject matter. Although, all modes of rhetoric are present in every act of communication, one often finds one or two modes of persuasion dominating in a particular context and ideology. For instance, in the case of Aristotle's center-Right rhetoric, the emphasis is on natural order, yet there is also a focus on ethos and pathos. In fact, I argue that ethos dominates authoritarian ideology, while logos is the main mode of modernity and liberal democratic ideology; furthermore, while pathos is often invoked by Leftist ideologies, libertarian ideology is mainly determined by a fourth form, which Aristotle will call in the *Poetics*, catharsis.[92] We can therefore understand a particular ideology by what mode of persuasion is the most prevalent.

A paradox of Aristotle's rhetoric is that he often sounds modern because of his stress on reason, universality, and science, yet due to his underlying investment in natural order, social hierarchy, and self-interest, these modern attributes are framed by a center-Right desire to see oneself as pure and innocent.[93] For example, the following passage could be seen as arguing for a modern concept of universal law; however, we must remember that Aristotle's culture only allowed certain groups of people to be covered by legal protections:

> If the written law tells against our case, clearly we must appeal to the universal law, and insist on its greater equity and justice. We must argue that the juror's oath "I will give my verdict according to my honest opinion" means that one will not simply follow the letter of the written law. We must urge that the principles of equity are permanent and changeless, and that the universal law does not change either, for it is the law of nature, whereas written laws often do change.
>
> (*R*: 59)

By arguing that the law should be universal, Aristotle anticipates the modern liberal democratic concept of equal justice; however, he ties this universality to an unchanging natural law. Thus, by naturalizing equality and justice, he removes them from the modern construction of a changeable, expanding system of justice.[94]

In terms of modernity, the universal has to be dynamic because it needs to be open to the inclusion of new groups. For instance, throughout the postmodern period, we have seen women, people of color, and the poor included into universalizing human rights.[95] On one level, modern law is universal since it is centered on equal protection and treatment, yet on another level, the universal has to remain open to being revised by new circumstances. Here we find the current conflict between originalists who believe that the constitution is based on unchanging natural law, and the contextualists, who affirm that the law must always take into account current circumstances.

To better understand the way that context and history shape ideology, I will examine in the next chapter Erich Fromm's *Escape from Freedom*. What is so important about this work is that it combines psychoanalysis and historical analysis in order to present a dialectical understanding of ideological formations. Moreover, Fromm helps us to understand the roots of authoritarian and libertarian ideologies from a conservative perspective.

Notes

1 Barnes, Jonathan (ed.). *The Cambridge companion to Aristotle*. Cambridge University Press, 1995. Hereafter cited as "*R*" in this chapter.
2 Nietzsche, Friedrich Wilhelm. *The genealogy of morals*. Boni & Liveright, 2017.
3 Simpson, Peter L. Phillips (ed.). *The politics of Aristotle*. University of North Carolina Press, 2000.
4 Ambler, Wayne. "Aristotle on nature and politics: The case of slavery." *Political Theory* 15.3 (1987): 390–410.
5 Smith, Nicholas D. "Aristotle's theory of natural slavery." *Phoenix* 37.2 (1983): 109–122.
6 Frank, Jill. "Citizens, slaves, and foreigners: Aristotle on human nature." *American Political Science Review* 98.1 (2004): 91–104.
7 Olson, Hope A. "Exclusivity, teleology and hierarchy: Our Aristotelean legacy." *Knowledge Organization* 26.2 (1999): 65–73.
8 Levin, Michael. "Natural subordination, Aristotle on." *Philosophy* 72.280 (1997): 241–257.
9 Reynolds, Nedra. "Ethos as location: New sites for understanding discursive authority." *Rhetoric Review* 11.2 (1993): 325–338.
10 Finlayson, Alan. "Ideology and political rhetoric." *The Oxford handbook of political ideologies* (2013): 197–213.
11 Leighton, Stephen. "Aristotle's account of anger: Narcissism and illusions of self-sufficiency." *Ratio* 15.1 (2002): 23–45.
12 Lindsay, Thomas K. "Was Aristotle racist, sexist, and anti-democratic? A review essay." *The Review of politics* 56.1 (1994): 127–151.
13 Cook, Kathleen C. "Sexual inequality in Aristotle's theories of reproduction and inheritance." In Julie K. Ward (ed.), *Feminism and ancient philosophy*. Routledge, 2019: 51–67.
14 Dea, Shannon. *Beyond the binary: Thinking about sex and gender*. Second edition. Broadview Press, 2023.
15 Mercer, Christia. "The philosophical roots of Western misogyny." *philosophical topics* 46.2 (2018): 183–208.
16 Fernandez, James W. "Rhetoric in the moral order: A critique of tropological approaches to culture." *Culture, rhetoric and the vicissitudes of life* (2009): 156–172.
17 Amussen, Susan D. "Social hierarchies." In Susan Doran and Norman Jones (eds.), *The Elizabethan world*. Routledge, 2014: 289–302.
18 Furley, David. "Aristotle the philosopher of nature." In David Furley (ed.), *Routledge history of philosophy*. Volume II. Routledge, 2003: 30–60.
19 Howell, Signe. "Nature in culture or culture in nature." In Philippe Descola and Gisli Palsson (eds.), *Nature and society: Anthropological perspectives*. Routledge, 1996: 127–144.
20 Thompson, Michael. "Socially viable ideas of nature: a cultural hypothesis." In Erik Baark and Uno Svedin (eds.), *Man, nature and technology: Essays on the role of ideological perceptions*. Palgrave Macmillan, 1988: 57–79.
21 Carbado, Devon W. "Racial naturalization." *American Quarterly* 57.3 (2005): 633–658.

22 Kullmann, Wolfgang. "Aristotle as a natural scientist." *Acta Classica: Proceedings of the Classical Association of South Africa* 34.1 (1991).

23 Vega, Jesús. "Aristotle on practical rules, universality, and the law." *The Threads of Natural Law: Unravelling a Philosophical Tradition.* Dordrecht: Springer Netherlands, 2012. 1–25.

24 Van Wees, Hans, and Nick Fisher. "The trouble with 'aristocracy'." In Nick Fisher and Hans van Wees, *"Aristocracy" in antiquity: Redefining Greek and Roman elites.* Classical Press of Wales, 2015: 1–57.

25 Mignolo, Walter, Stuart Elden, and Eduardo Mendieta. *The darker side of the Enlightenment: Reading Kant's geography.* State University of New York Press, 2011.

26 Kolm, Serge-Christophe. *Modern theories of justice.* MIT Press, 2002.

27 Meikle, Scott. "Aristotle on equality and market exchange." *The Journal of Hellenic Studies* 111 (1991): 193–196.

28 Moss, Jessica. "Right reason in Plato and Aristotle: On the meaning of logos." *Phronesis* 59.3 (2014): 181–230.

29 Konrádová, Veronika. "Public reasoning and the role of logos in Gorgias and Aristotle." *ΠΗΓΗ/FONS* 6 (2021): 15–29.

30 Galston, Miriam. "Taking Aristotle seriously: Republican-oriented legal theory and the moral foundation of deliberative democracy." *California Law Review* 82 (1994): 329.

31 Bloom, Paul. "Empathy and its critics." In Troy DuJardin and M. David Eckel (eds.), *Faith, hope, and love: The theological virtues and their opposites.* Springer, 2022: 177–187.

32 McCormack, Krista C. "Ethos, pathos, and logos: The benefits of Aristotelian rhetoric in the courtroom." *Washington University Jurisprudence Review* 7 (2014): 131.

33 Samuels, Robert. *Žižek and the rhetorical unconscious: Global politics, philosophy, and subjectivity.* Springer, 2020.

34 Kinneavy, James L., and Catherine R. Eskin. "Kairos in Aristotle's rhetoric." *Written Communication* 17.3 (2000): 432–444.

35 Crivelli, Paolo. *Aristotle on truth.* Cambridge University Press, 2004.

36 Finnis, John. *Natural law and natural rights.* Oxford University Press, 2011.

37 Strang, Lee J. *Originalism's promise: A natural law account of the American Constitution.* Cambridge University Press, 2019.

38 Mikhail, John. "Does originalism have a natural law problem?." *Law and History Review* 39.2 (2021): 361–367.

39 Olson, R. Michael. "Aristotle on God: Divine nous as unmoved mover." In Jeanine Diller and Asa Kasher (eds.), *Models of God and alternative ultimate realities.* Springer, 2012: 101–109.

40 Long, Christopher P. *Aristotle on the nature of truth.* Cambridge University Press, 2010.

41 Rivers, Nathaniel A., and Maarten Derksen. "Ecologies of deception in psychology and rhetoric." *Quarterly Journal of Speech* 101.4 (2015): 633–654.

42 Ryan, Eugene E. "Aristotle's rhetoric and ethics and the ethos of society." *Greek, Roman, and Byzantine Studies* 13.3 (1972): 291–308.

43 Shils, Edward. "The academic ethos." *The American Scholar* (1978): 165–190.

44 Schendzielorz, Cornelia, and Martin Reinhart. "Relating democratic and scientific ethos in academic self-governance." *Serendipities: Journal for the Sociology and History of the Social Sciences* 6.2 (2022): 1–20.

45 Ober, Josiah. "Aristotle's political sociology: Class, status, and order in the politics." In Carnes Lord and David K. O'Connor (eds)., *Essays on the foundations of Aristotelian political science.* University of California Press, 1991: 112–135.

46 Braet, Antoine C. "Ethos, pathos and logos in Aristotle's *Rhetoric*: A re-examination." *Argumentation* 6 (1992): 307–320.
47 Samuels, Robert. *Žižek and the rhetorical unconscious: Global politics, philosophy, and subjectivity.* Springer, 2020.
48 Samuels, Robert. "Pathos, hysteria, and the Left." In Robert Samuels, *Žižek and the rhetorical unconscious: Global politics, philosophy, and subjectivity.* Springer, 2020: 33–47.
49 Mulhern, M. M. "Aristotle on universality and necessity." *Logique et Analyse* 12.47 (1969): 288–299.
50 Madden, Edward H. "Aristotle's treatment of probability and signs." *Philosophy of Science* 24.2 (1957): 167–172.
51 Sbisà, Marina. "Speech act theory." In Jef Verschueren and Jan-Ola Östman (eds.), *Key notions for pragmatics.* John Benjamins, 2009: 229–244.
52 Short, Bryan C. "The temporality of rhetoric." *Rhetoric Review*7.2 (1989): 367–379.
53 Smith, Joseph H. "The pleasure principle." *The International Journal of Psycho-Analysis* 58 (1977): 1.
54 Samuels, Robert. "Catharsis: The politics of enjoyment." Robert Samuels, *Žižek and the rhetorical unconscious: Global politics, philosophy, and subjectivity.* Springer, 2020: 7–31.
55 Annas, Julia. "Aristotle on pleasure and goodness." In Amélie Oksenberg Rorty (ed.), *Essays on Aristotle's ethics.* University of California Press, 1980: 285–299.
56 Annas, Julia. "Aristotle on pleasure and goodness." In Amélie Oksenberg Rorty (ed.), *Essays on Aristotle's ethics.* University of California Press, 1980: 285–299.
57 Rorty, Amelie Oksenberg. "The place of pleasure in Aristotle's ethics." *Mind* 83.332 (1974): 481–497.
58 Cruz Ortiz de Landázuri, Manuel M. "Virtue without pleasure? Aristotle and the joy of a noble life." *Acta Philosophica: Rivista Internazionale di Filosofia* 23.1 (2014): 89–100.
59 Hall, Edith. "'Master of those who know': Aristotle as role model for the twenty-first century academician." *European Review* 25.1 (2017): 3–19.
60 Bevan, David L. "Inheritance and the distribution of wealth." *Economica* 46.184 (1979): 381–402.
61 Donohue, Brian. "Beauty and motivation in Aristotle." *Quaestiones Disputatae* 6.2 (2016): 26–43.
62 Sylvester, Charles. "The classical idea of leisure: Cultural ideal or class prejudice?" *Leisure Sciences* 21.1 (1999): 3–16.
63 Scheurich, James J. "Social relativism:(not quite) a postmodernist epistemology." In James J. Scheurich, *Research method in the postmodern.* Routledge, 2014: 29–60.
64 Norris, Pippa, and Ronald Inglehart. *Cultural backlash: Trump, Brexit, and authoritarian populism.* Cambridge University Press, 2019.
65 Rosler, Andrés. *Political authority and obligation in Aristotle.* Oxford University Press, 2005.
66 Schaper, Eva. "Aristotle's catharsis and aesthetic pleasure." *The Philosophical Quarterly* 18.71 (1968): 131–143.
67 Berczeller, Eva. "The 'aesthetic feeling' and Aristotle's catharsis theory." *The Journal of Psychology* 65.2 (1967): 261–271.
68 Samuels, Robert. "Catharsis: The politics of enjoyment." In Robert Samuels, *Žižek and the rhetorical unconscious: Global politics, philosophy, and subjectivity.* Springer, 2020: 7–31.
69 Wheeler, Marcus. "Aristotle's analysis of the nature of political struggle." *The American Journal of Philology* 72.2 (1951): 145–161.

70 Brzechczyn, Krzysztof. "Varieties of idealization and strategies of modification of social theory. The case of the totalitarian syndrome." *Człowiek i Społeczeństwo* 34 (2012): 235–247.
71 Williamson, Colwyn, and Stuart Brown. "The social order and the natural order." *Proceedings of the Aristotelian Society, Supplementary Volumes* 52 (1978): 109–141.
72 McGrade, Arthur Stephen. "Aristotle's place in the history of natural rights." *The Review of Metaphysics* (1996): 803–829.
73 Spiegel, John P. "Violence and the social order." *Zygon* 4.3 (1969): 222–237.
74 West, William N. "Repeating staging meaning between Aristotle and Freud." *SubStance* 28.2 (1999): 138–158.
75 Lott, Micah. "Why be a good human being? Natural goodness, reason, and the authority of human nature." *Philosophia* 42 (2014): 761–777.
76 Parrott, W. Gerrod. "The social construction of emotions." In Bo Allesøe Christensen (ed.), *The second cognitive revolution: A tribute to Rom Harré*. Springer, 2019: 131–139.
77 Modell, Arnold H. "Emotional memory, metaphor, and meaning." *Psychoanalytic Inquiry* 25.4 (2005): 555–568.
78 Deigh, John. "Emotions: the legacy of James and Freud." *The International Journal of Psychoanalysis* 82.6 (2001): 1247–1256.
79 Reginster, Bernard. "Nietzsche on pleasure and power." *Philosophical Topics* 33.2 (2005): 161–191.
80 Samuels, Robert. "Beyond Hillary Clinton: Obsessional narcissism and the failure of the liberal class." In Robert Samuels, *Psychoanalyzing the Left and Right after Donald Trump: Conservatism, liberalism, and neoliberal populisms*. Springer, 2016: 31–59.
81 Samuels, Robert. "(Liberal) narcissism." In Yannis Stavrakakis (ed.), *Routledge handbook of psychoanalytic political theory*. Routledge, 2019: 151–161.
82 Betsakos, Vassilios. "Imitation and learning, Learning and pleasure, Aristotle, *Poetics* 4." *Dia-noesis: A Journal of Philosophy* 7 (2019): 7–28.
83 Gonzalez, Francisco J. "Aristotle on pleasure and perfection." *Phronesis* 36.2 (1991): 141–159.
84 Benedikter, Roland, Katja Siepmann, and Fabian Kupper. "The cultural dimension: A nation in search of identity between the competing narratives of the 'center-Right' and the 'center-Left'." In Roland Benedikter and Katja Siepmann (eds.), *Chile in transition: Prospects and challenges for Latin America's forerunner of development*. Springer, 2015: 35–77.
85 Freud, Sigmund. *On narcissism: An introduction*. Read Books, 2014.
86 Stewart, Matthew. *The 9.9 percent: The new aristocracy that is entrenching inequality and warping our culture*. Simon and Schuster, 2022.
87 Goodrich, Peter. "Law and modernity." *The Modern Law Review* 49.5 (1986): 545–559.
88 Olson, Hope A. "Exclusivity, teleology and hierarchy: Our Aristotelean legacy." *Knowledge Organization* 26.2 (1999): 65–73.
89 Samuels, Robert. *Teaching writing, rhetoric, and reason at the globalizing university*. Routledge, 2020.
90 Longaker, Mark Garrett. "Idealism and early-American rhetoric." *Rhetoric Society Quarterly* 36.3 (2006): 281–308.
91 Beale, Walter H. *A pragmatic theory of rhetoric*. SIU Press, 1987.
92 Samuels, Robert. *Žižek and the rhetorical unconscious: Global politics, philosophy, and subjectivity*. Springer Nature, 2020.
93 Brooks, David. "Bobos in paradise: The new upper class and how they got there." In David Grusky and Jasmine Hill (eds.), *Inequality in the 21st century: A reader*. Routledge, 2018: 95–99.

94 Chernilo, Daniel. *The natural law foundations of modern social theory: A quest for universalism*. Cambridge University Press, 2013.
95 Brysk, Alison. "Expanding human rights." In Alison Brysk (ed.), *Expanding human rights*. Edward Elgar Publishing, 2017. 3–10.

Chapter 6

Erich Fromm and the Social Construction of Ideology and Subjectivity

Through its combination of Marx and Freud, Erich Fromm's *Escape from Freedom* presents a historical account of the development of distinct ideologies and the relational desires driving them.[1] Thus, in opposition to Aristotle's naturalization of social hierarchies and belief systems, Fromm attempts to show how economics, history, and psychology shape what ideologies people support. Moreover, unlike the current move to base ideological commitment on the workings of individual brains, Fromm uses a social mode of psychoanalysis to expose the underlying mental processes that define why we believe in specific ideological formations.[2]

A Conservative Model

Fromm frames his analysis of ideology by taking a historical perspective on the development of particular social structures and belief systems:

> What characterizes medieval in contrast – to modern society is its lack of individual freedom. Everybody in the earlier period was chained to his role in the social order. A man had little chance to move socially from one class to another, he was hardly able to move even geographically from one town or from one country to another. With few exceptions he had to stay where he was born. The artisan had to sell at a certain price and the peasant at a certain place, the market of the town.
>
> (*EF*: 57)

Although Fromm focuses on the distinction between Medieval and modern societies, what he is really targeting is the opposition between a traditional, rigid, unchanging social hierarchy and a capitalist society shaped by class and economic mobility.[3] Moreover, he emphasizes that the loss of a traditional social order results in a sense of loneliness and anxiety for the free individual.[4] In other words, from his conservative perspective, the problem with modernity is that it liberates the individual from any pre-established order or meaning, and this loss of traditional ideology produces a libertarian

DOI: 10.4324/9781003773948-6

subject who instead of enjoying their freedom feels an intense sense of anxiety.

One of the problems with Fromm's analysis here is that he tends to confuse libertarian ideology with conservative ideology because instead of recognizing the pleasure of the desire for freedom, he focuses on the anxiety caused by a loss of pre-established order.[5] As we learn from Freud, anxiety is generated when a person cannot predict what will happen next on a mental level, and so what conservatives desire is to return to some type of traditional order where everything is structured by a predetermined meaning.[6] Thus, conservatives call for a return to the past because they experience anxiety when they are alone and without order and meaning.[7]

In his description of what I have been calling traditional ideology, Fromm highlights the relational desire for a fixed social order:

> But although a person was not free in the modem sense, neither was he alone and isolated. In having a distinct, unchangeable, and unquestionable place in the social world from the moment of birth, man was rooted in a structuralized whole, and thus life had a meaning which left no place, and no need, for doubt. A person was identical with his role in society; he was a peasant, an artisan, a knight, and not an individual who happened to have this or that occupation. The social order was conceived as a natural order, and being a definite part of it gave a feeling of security and of belonging. There was comparatively little competition. One was born into a certain economic position which guaranteed a livelihood determined by tradition, just as it carried economic obligations to those higher in the social hierarchy.
>
> (*EF*: 58)

What helps to define tradition here is the idea that one is born into a world that is already organized, and every social subject has a defined place within the social hierarchy.[8] Thus, in opposition to the modern notion of economic and class mobility, this pre-modern order values stability and predictability over individual freedom.[9] In turn, when this pre-established order is lost, one suffers from the anxiety of not knowing their place or understanding how the world works. In order to control this anxiety, the conservative desires protection through the return to a stable and predictable world.[10]

What Fromm does not clearly distinguish, however, is the difference between traditional ideology and the authoritarian ideology delivered by Christianity: While tradition is centered on social and natural order, religious fundamentalists are seeking salvation by submitting to a higher power.[11] For Fromm, one of the main ways that Christianity gained believers was by not only offering a new community but also providing an explanation and solution to suffering, guilt, and shame: "There was much suffering and pain, but there was also the Church which made this suffering more tolerable by explaining it as a result of the sin of Adam and the individual sins of each person" (*EF*: 58). On the most basic level, Christianity offers salvation by presenting a cause for suffering and sin, which also turns out to be the solution:

> the Church fostered a sense of guilt, it also assured the individual of her unconditional love to all her children and offered a way to acquire the conviction of being forgiven and loved by God. The relationship to God was more one of confidence and love than of doubt and fear. Just as a peasant and a town dweller rarely went beyond the limits of the small geographical area which was theirs, so the universe was limited and simple to understand. The earth and man were its center, heaven or hell was the future place of life, and all actions from birth to death were transparent in their causal interrelation.
>
> (*EF*: 59)

To the traditional social order, monotheistic religions offer a single power and explanation by establishing an imaginary relationship between the believer and a higher power.[12] As we shall see, this type of ideology offers salvation through idealization and submission: Since one believes that a single force controls everything, and that force loves and forgives one, all guilt and shame is removed, yet the cost is that one also has to stop testing reality or thinking in a critical fashion.[13] Moreover, Fromm's central theory is that this desire for salvation results in an escape from freedom as the individual gives up their own liberty and reason in order to eliminate negative feelings about the self.[14] After all, if one transfers power and responsibility to an all-powerful being, then one cannot be held responsible for one's own faulty actions and anti-social desires. As we shall see, this combination of submission to a higher power and the release from responsibility defines the essence of authoritarian ideology.

The Rise of Capitalism and the Center-Left

Following Marx, Fromm insists that it is capitalism itself that undermined traditional and authoritarian ideologies because this economic system focused on the desire and actions of the isolated individual:

> The structure of society and the personality of man changed in the late Middle Ages. The unity and centralization of medieval society became weaker. Capital, individual economic initiative and competition grew in importance; a new moneyed class developed. A growing individualism was noticeable in all social classes and affected all spheres of human activity, taste, fashion, art, philosophy, and theology.
>
> (*EF*: 60)

Just as Marx argues that exchange value melted away all solid premodern beliefs and institutions, Fromm posits that modern capitalism undermined traditional and authoritarian ideologies by placing the focus of society on individual economic initiative, competition, and money.[15] In other words, the rise of a libertarian ideology destabilized the premodern traditional and authoritarian social order, which resulted in the production of anxiety for the conservative subject.

Although Fromm tends to affirm a Marxist conception of ideology and history, there is an underlying conservative aspect to his discourse because he constantly returns to the notion that the main effect of modernity was to leave individuals alone and anxious:

> They were more free, but they were also more alone. They used their power and wealth to squeeze the last ounce of pleasure out of life; but in doing so, they had to use ruthlessly every means, from physical torture to psychological manipulation, to rule over the masses and to check their competitors within their own class. All human relationships were poisoned by this fierce life-and-death struggle for the maintenance of power and wealth. Solidarity with one's fellow men—or at least with the members of one's own class—was replaced by a cynical detached attitude; other individuals were looked upon as "objects" to be used and manipulated, or they were ruthlessly destroyed if it suited one's own ends.
>
> (*EF*: 65)

In many ways, what Fromm is describing is the conservative reaction to libertarian ideology. While the political Right celebrates the freedom of the individual to act on his impulses and desires, the conservative laments the loss of social order and meaning.[16] Furthermore, Fromm locates in libertarian social relations an underlying cynicism since everyone becomes an object for everyone else's manipulation.[17] In this form of nihilism, people do not believe in anything except the need to act on their drives as they imagine that everyone else is doing the same thing.[18]

With Fromm's critique of modern capitalism and the libertarian Right, we discover that the relational desire for freedom can result in an insatiable drive:

> The individual was absorbed by a passionate egocentricity, an insatiable greed for power and wealth. As a result of all this, the successful individual's relation to his own self, his sense of security and confidence were poisoned too. His own self became as much an object of manipulation to him as other persons had become.
>
> (*EF*: 65)

From Fromm's perspective, libertarian ideology not only functions to objectify others, but it also turns the self into an object of manipulation.[19] Thus, in opposition to the center-Left, narcissistic desire for having the ideal self admired, the libertarian drive results in self-objectification: The more one acts on one's selfish desires, the more one becomes an object of one's drives.[20]

While much of Fromm's analysis is accurate, he tends to confuse the liberal ideology of modern science and democratic equality with the libertarian emphasis on capitalistic individualism.[21]He also frames this analysis through the use of a conservative ideology where the emphasis is on the anxiety and loneliness of the isolated individual:

> We have reasons to doubt whether the powerful masters of Renaissance capitalism were as happy and as secure as they are often pictured. It seems that the new freedom brought two things to them: an increased feeling of strength and at the same time an increased isolation, doubt, scepticism, and-resulting from all these-anxiety. It is the same contradiction that we find in the philosophic writings of the humanists.
>
> (*EF*: 65)

Although the modern liberal philosophers like Descartes did use doubt as a way to seek out truth, their discourse tended to replace the isolated individual with the universal subject of science and democratic law.[22] In other terms, the way that they sought to overcome anxiety was by affirming the need for scientific evidence and impersonal universality.

Fromm adds that the narcissistic desire for admiration can also be a way of overcoming a sense of insecurity and isolation that comes from the loss of the traditional social order:

> This underlying insecurity resulting from the position of an isolated individual in a hostile world tends to explain the genesis of a character trait which was, as Burckhardt has pointed out, characteristic of the individual of the Renaissance and not present, at least in the same intensity, in the member of the medieval social structure: his passionate craving for fame.
>
> (*EF*: 66)

While for the conservative subject, anxiety is derived from the need to protected against unknows risks and dangers, the desire for fame and admiration helps the center-Left narcissist to regain a sense of identity and purpose:

> If the meaning of life has become doubtful, if one's relations to others and to oneself do not offer security, then fame is one means to silence one's doubts. It has a function to be compared with that of the Egyptian pyramids or the Christian faith in immortality: it elevates one's individual life from its limitations and instability to the plane of indestructibility; if one's name is known to one's contemporaries and if one can

> hope that it will last for centuries, then one's life has meaning and significance by this very reflection of it in the judgments of others. It is obvious that this solution ·of individual insecurity was only possible for a social group whose members possessed the actual means of gaining fame.
> (*EF*: 66)

This use of fame to overcome insecurity relates to the notion that underlying the narcissist's desire for admiration, there is a repressed sense of insecurity.[23]

From Fromm's perspective, this quest for fame was partially enabled by the lost connection between economic activity and morality:

> There is no place in medieval theory for economic activity which is not related to a moral end, and to found a science of society upon the assumption that the appetite for economic gain is a constant and measurable force, to be accepted like other natural forces, as an inevitable and self-evident datum, would have appeared to the medieval thinker as hardly less irrational and less immoral than to make the premise of social philosophy the unrestrained operation of such necessary human attributes as pugnacity and the sexual instinct ...
> (*EF*: 71)

According to this theory, in the feudal period, economics and morality were seen as belonging to the same natural order, and therefore, it was impossible to see the drive for more money as a purely individualistic desire without social consequences. In fact, Luther railed against the growing power of capitalism to reshape all aspects of life:

> The indignation and rage of the small merchant against the monopolies was given eloquent expression by Luther in his pamphlet "On Trading and Usury," printed in 1524. "They have all commodities under their control and practise without concealment all the tricks that have been mentioned; they raise and lower prices as they please For and oppress and ruin all the small merchants, as the pike the little fish in the water, just as though they were lords over God's creatures and free from all the laws of faith and love."
> (*EF*: 74–75)

In combining authoritarian, traditional, and conservative ideologies in the moral fight against capitalism, Luther's religious politics shows how the feudal period had not yet fully given into the libertarian power of markets to reshape life.[24]

With the rise of modern capitalism, and the loss of the old premodern social order, a new mode of individualism was born, which reveals the essence of the libertarian Right:

> With the rise of capitalism these medieval principles gave way more and more to a principle of individualistic enterprise. Each individual must go ahead and try his luck. He had to swim or to sink. Others were not allied with him in a common enterprise, they became competitors, and often he was confronted with the choice of destroying them or being destroyed.
>
> (*EF*: 79)

Here we encounter the foundations of libertarian ideology and its relation to the borderline personality: In a world that is structured by competing individuals with no higher beliefs, everyone is motivated to act on their own drives while denying the need to share with others or regulate the self.[25] As a cynical ideology, the relational desire for freedom and pleasure is tied to the fantasy of a constant-sum game where either one has the object of desire or the other holds the envied object.[26]

One of the side-effects of modern capitalism is that it tended to undermine the old traditional order:

> It freed man from the regimentation of the corporative system; it allowed him to stand on his own feet and to try his luck. He became the master of his fate, his was the risk, his the gain. Individual effort could lead him to success and economic independence. Money became the great equalizer of man and proved to be more powerful than birth and caste.
>
> (*EF*: 80)

In this form of economic competition and Right-wing ideology, it is up to the individual to sink or swim, and all cooperation is denied.[27]

According to Fromm's conservative perspective, the end result of the growing dominance of modern capitalism and libertarian ideology is an increased sense of insecurity and anxiety:

> Paradise is lost for good, the individual stands alone and faces the world-a stranger thrown into a limitless and threatening world. The new freedom is bound to create a deep feeling of insecurity, powerlessness, doubt, aloneness, and anxiety. These feelings must be alleviated if the individual is to function successfully.
>
> (*EF*: 81)

While conservatives focus on the loss of social order and the increase in anxiety due to insecurity, for the libertarian capitalists, this anxiety is released through the pleasure of consumption and the denial of social regulation and morality.[28]

The Psychopathology of Political Ideologies

It is vital to stress that in Freud's conception of the different agencies of the human mind, he separates the internalized social morality (the super-ego) from the pursuit of pleasure (the id) and sees the ego as being attacked by the conscience and the drives.[29] Anxiety is then generated when not only is the social order suspended, but there is also no way to overcome a loss of protection through the idealization of some saving Other (the ego ideal).[30] Likewise, as we saw in the structure of narcissism, the individual seeks to escape anxiety and the drives by establishing an ideal ego, which both conforms to social morality and signals its exceptional status to itself and others.[31] Moreover, in addition to these five agencies (the id, ego, super-ego, the ego-ideal, and the ideal ego), Freud adds that the reality-ego must use reason and reality testing to discover both internal and external truth.[32]

If we now attach each of these different internal mental agencies to specific ideologies and pathologies, we find that traditional culture is reliant on a psychotic investment in the super-ego, while libertarian ideology feeds off of the dominance of the id.[33] In turn, it is the vulnerable conservative ego that feels attacked by the id, the super-ego, and the lack of a saving ego-ideal, while authoritarians seek to escape guilt, shame, and anxiety by idealizing the Other (the ego-ideal) and suspending their own reality-testing ego (the reality-ego).[34] Finally with the ideology of center-Left narcissism, the ideal ego represses the id and conforms to the super-ego on a superficial and ironic level.[35]

The final agency that Freud attaches to psychopathology is his theory of the symptom, which is focused on the detection of unpleasure.[36] In the structure of hysteria, the expression of suffering through symptoms is used to both gain a sense of identity and to influence others through the production of guilt within a victim complex.[37] In turning real and imagined suffering into an identity and a demand made to others, the essence of Leftist protest and the desire for accommodation is revealed.[38] In many ways, the necessary development of the postmodern welfare state embodies this hysterical desire for accommodation as the disempowered and disadvantaged seek out special treatment.[39]

What is then missing from most accounts of ideology is an understanding of the different types of mental agencies and psychopathologies that dominate in particular belief systems and social structures. In fact, Fromm points to this relation between ideology and psychopathology when he attempts to tie subjective motivations to particular social doctrines:

> What the psychological analysis of doctrines can show is the subjective motivations which make a person aware of certain problems and make him seek for answers in certain directions. Any kind of thought, true or false, if it is more than a superficial conformance with conventional

> ideas, is motivated by the subjective needs and interests of the person who is thinking.
>
> (*EF*: 82)

This indication of the importance specific subjective motivations play in the affirmation of particular ideologies can be related to my focus on relational desires.[40]

Fromm is also aware that the relation between subjectivity and society often is determined by psychopathology:

> The influence of any doctrine or idea depends on the ·extent to which it appeals to psychic needs in the character structure of those to whom it is addressed. Only if the idea answers powerful psychological needs of certain social groups will it become a potent force in history.
>
> (*EF*: 83)

Here, the psychopathology of political ideology is most apparent since Fromm realizes that the influence of any ideology rests on the way that it caters to particular subjective needs, and these needs are themselves determined by how a specific mental agency and pathology dominates in particular individuals.[41]

As Fromm indicates, psychopathology not only explains why people gravitate towards specific ideologies, it also points to the psychology of the leaders of social groups:

> Both problems, the psychology of the leader and that of his followers, are, of course, closely linked with each other. If the same ideas appeal to them their character structure must be similar in important aspects. Aside from factors such as the special talent for thinking and action on the part of the leader, his character structure will usually exhibit in a more extreme and clear-cut way the particular personality structure of those to whom his doctrines appeal; he can arrive at a clearer and more outspoken formulation of certain ideas for which his followers are already prepared psychologically.
>
> (*EF*: 83)

Fromm is arguing that the leaders of a particular ideological group represent an extreme form of the psychopathology of the members, but it should be clear that this is not always the case.[42] For instance, one of Freud's key insights into authoritarian ideology is that the followers desire salvation through idealization, while the leader desires freedom and power.[43] Thus, people may identify with the leader who is free to act on his drives without restriction, yet what determines their submission is their desire to escape freedom in order to escape responsibility.

Luther and Subjective Submission

In terms of his discussion of Luther and his submissive followers, Fromm indicates that the psychopathology of the leader can be highly conflicted and narcissistic: "He hated others, especially the 'rabble,' he hated himself, he hated life; and out of all this hatred came a passionate and desperate striving to be loved" (*EF*: 84). On the one hand, Luther has a great desire to be loved and protected, but on the other hand, this desire was driven by a high level of self-hatred.[44] In this narcissistic structure, the relational call for admiration seeks to shout down the disgust caused by the id:

> Luther's theology gave expression to the feelings of the middle class which, fighting against the authority of the Church and resenting the new moneyed class, felt threatened by rising capitalism and overcome by a feeling of powerlessness and individual insignificance.
>
> (*EF*: 92)

Here, the middle-class is located in a middle position between authoritarian and libertarian ideologies: By rebelling against Christianity and resenting the winners of the capitalist system, these centrists were attracted to Luther's own divided discourse.[45]

What we then find in the development of Protestant religion and ideology is a belief system and subjectivity shaped by the focus on the individual who is caught between idealized authority and de-stabilizing capitalism:

> This aspect points out that he gave man independence in religious matters; that he deprived the Church of her authority and gave it to the individual; that his concept of faith and salvation is one of subjective individual experience, in which all responsibility is with the individual and none with an authority which could give him what he cannot obtain himself. There are good reasons to praise this side of Luther's and Calvin's doctrines, since they are one—source of the development of political and spiritual freedom in modem society; a development which, especially in Anglo-Saxon countries, is inseparably connected with the ideas of Puritanism.
>
> (*EF*: 93)

The important move that Fromm finds in the formation of Protestantism is the notion that the desire for salvation had become individualized as one sought to be saved on a personal level and not through submission to a collective organization.[46] As a central aspect of center-Left ideology and middle-class narcissistic subjectivity, the personalization of religion and authority points to the internalization and neutralization of the ego-ideal as a source for self-idealization.[47] While Fromm sees this transformation as a move towards greater freedom and individualism, it should be clear that this structure can lead to a repressed investment in libertarian ideology. As the ideal ego seeks to be admired by the Other in an act of superficial virtue signaling, the underlying desire is for the freedom to act on one's desires without regulation.[48]

As Luther's discourse reveals, underlying this center-Left mentality is a belief in the inherent sinfulness of human desire: "Luther assumed the existence of an innate evilness in man's nature, which directs his will for evil and makes it impossible for any man to perform any good deed on the basis of his nature. Man has an evil and vicious nature" (*EF*: 93). Similar to Freud's theory that behind every altruistic act, there is an underlying anti-social hostility, Fromm points to Luther's belief that every person is evil by nature.[49] In fact, Freud told the narcissistic and obsessive Rat Man that his morality is conscious, but his immorality remains unconscious.[50] Since the center-Left narcissist wants to maintain an idealized self-image, it is necessary to hide the id, yet with Luther, we find a leader who wants to expose selfish drives in order to get people to freely submit to a higher power.

Through the manipulation of self-hatred and traditional morality, Luther desired to enforce the submission to an idealized higher power, yet he wanted people to do it in such a way that they were able to maintain a sense of individual freedom and autonomy:

> This conviction of man's rottenness and powerlessness to do anything good on his own merits is one essential condition of God's grace. Only if man humiliates himself and demolishes his individual will and pride will God's grace descend upon him. "For God wants to save us not by our own but by extraneous (*fremde*) justice and wisdom, by a justice that does not come from ourselves and does not originate in ourselves but comes to us from somewhere else … That is, a justice must be taught that comes exclusively from the outside and is entirely alien to ourselves."
>
> (*EF*: 94)

Luther's ideology is therefore inherently contradictory since he wants people to submit unconditionally to an external power, yet he also thinks people should act freely as individuals.[51] This contradiction relates to the problem of how one can combine a theory of predestination with one of human choice.[52] After all, if we are all fated to either go to heaven or hell, why should we try to act in a moral way? The solution that Luther and other Protestants propose to this conflict is to argue that the way that you know you have been chosen is by being rewarded for your present good work.[53]

The Protestant reconciliation of predetermination and human freedom points to a fundamental concern of all ideologies, which is how do you deal with the unresolvable conflict between society and the individual. In fact, this conflict is the primal driving force behind Freud's entire project since he accepts that it is impossible to ever fully overcome it.[54] However, for Luther, the key move is to separate our strict obedience to an imagined higher power from our freedom in relation to other people:

> Luther declares that if one does not like "to leave out this theme (of free will) altogether (which would be most safe and also most religious) we may, nevertheless, with a good conscience teach that it be used so far as to allow man a 'free will,' not in respect of those who are above him, but in respect only of those beings who are below him ... God-ward man has no 'free will,' but is a captive, slave, and servant either to the will of God or to the will of Satan."
>
> (*EF*: 95)

Caught between the blind submission to a higher power or the domination by uncontrollable drives, the center-Left narcissist combines together a superficial conformity to social morality with a repressed sense of anti-social freedom.[55] In this form of the as-if subject, one becomes shaped by unconscious thoughts, feelings, and behaviors.[56]

For Fromm, Luther's twisted ideology was itself not successful in alleviating the anxiety of the modern man who was confronted with the loss of the traditional social order through the growing dominance of capitalist ideology:

> The doctrines that man was a powerless tool in God's hands and fundamentally evil, that his only task was to resign to the will of God, that God could save him as the result of an incomprehensible act of justice-these doctrines were not the definite answer a man was to give who was so much driven by despair, anxiety, and doubt and at the same time by such an ardent wish for certainty as Luther.
>
> (*EF*: 95)

The only solution to this profound anxiety driven by insecurity could be an affirmation of a transcendent faith:

> He eventually found the answer for his doubts. In 1518 a sudden revelation came to him. Man cannot be saved on the basis of his virtues; he should not even meditate whether or not his works were well pleasing to God; but he can have certainty of his salvation if he has faith.
>
> (*EF*: 95)

The underlying desire for salvation could only be resolved through a leap of faith, and in this structure, it did not matter if one acted in a virtuous way or not.[57]

Automaton or Authoritarian

At the end of his work, Fromm affirms that modern man is often forced between acting like a social automaton or submitting to an authoritarian ideology:

> in discussing the psychological results we have shown that this powerlessness leads either to the kind of escape that we find in the authoritarian character, or else to a compulsive conforming in the process of which the isolated individual becomes an automaton, loses his self, and yet at the same time consciously conceives of himself as free and subject only to himself.
>
> (*EF*: 266)

In the latter type of subjectivity, we see the essence of center-Left narcissism since what structures this ideology and psychopathology is a contradictory combination of conformity and autonomy.[58]

Fromm's main solution to how to deal with the dominate ideologies of his time is to focus on the need to use therapy and education to increase the independence and spontaneity of each individual: "This is not to say that training must inevitably lead to suppression of spontaneity—if the real aim of education is to further the inner independence and individuality of the child, its growth and integrity" (*EF*: 267). This focus on the ideals of independence and spontaneity may appear to follow Freud's theory of psychoanalytic treatment; however, it should be clear that Freud always sought to balance the needs of the individual with the role of society in regulating sex and violence. In other words, Freud does not prioritize a libertarian ideology since he realizes that there is a fundamental, unresolvable conflict between the self and society.[59]

To better understand the Freudian theory of ideology and globalism, I examine in the next chapter, the foundations of psychoanalytic social theory. Instead of simply favoring one ideology over the other, we shall see why it is necessary to distinguish and balance the distinct relational desires that shape our belief systems. While it is clear that Freud privileges modern science and reason as the keys to civilizational progress, his work offers an integrated approach to the eight central ideologies that structure global politics today.

Notes

1 Fromm, Erich. *Escape from freedom*. Holt, 1969. Hereafter cited as "*EF*" in this chapter.
2 Ingleby, David. "Psychoanalysis and ideology." In John M. Broughton (ed.), *Critical theories of psychological development*. Springer, 1987: 177–210.
3 Gregg, Samuel. "End of a myth: Max Weber, capitalism, and the medieval order." *Journal des conomistes et des tudes Humaines* 13.2 (2003).

4 Bendle, Mervyn F. "Erich Fromm and the age of anxiety." *Quadrant* 57.10 (2013): 66–72.
5 Maciel, Fabrício. "Erich Fromm and the culture of contemporary capitalism." *Fromm Forum* 23 (2019).
6 Svenaeus, Fredrik. "Freud's philosophy of the uncanny." *The Scandinavian Psychoanalytic Review* 22.2 (1999): 239–254.
7 Castano, Emanuele, et al. "Ideology, fear of death, and death anxiety." *Political Psychology* 32.4 (2011): 601–621.
8 Žižek, Slavoj. "The structure of domination today: A Lacanian view." *Studies in East European Thought* 56.4 (2004): 383–403.
9 Lopez, Julia Costa. "The premodern world." In Mlada Bukovansky, Edward Keene, Christian Reus-Smit, and Maja Spanu (eds.), *The Oxford handbook of history and international relations*. Oxford University Press, 2023: 395–409.
10 Söllner, Alfons. "Anxiety and politics: Neo-conservatism and critical theory." *Telos* 60 (1984): 129–132.
11 Freud, Sigmund. *Moses and monotheism*. Sanzani Edizioni, 2023.
12 Wilson, Henry S. "Salvation in world religions." *Mission Studies* 19.1 (2002): 108–135.
13 Freud, Sigmund. *The future of an illusion*. Broadview Press, 2012.
14 Akot, Bulent. "The perspective of psychological freedom and avoiding freedom according to Erich Fromm." *Hamdard Islamicus* 43.2 (2020).
15 Marx, Karl, and Friedrich Engels. "The communist manifesto." In Terence Ball, Richard Dagger, Daniel I. O'Neill, and Jennet Kirkpatrick (eds.), *Ideals and ideologies: A Reader*. Routledge, 2019: 243–255.
16 Kawabata, Toyo. "Anxiety in the capitalism of late modernity." *Emancipations* 2.2 (2023).
17 Macey, Jonathan R. "Cynicism and trust in politics and constitutional theory." *Cornell Law Review* 87 (2001): 280.
18 Barnes, Will. Liberal cynicism, its dangers, & a cure. Dissertation, University of New Mexico, 2018.
19 Thistlethwaite, Max. The mourning of lost autonomy: a philosophical and psychoanalytic critique on the objectification of fantasy. Dissertation, Brunel University, London, 2017.
20 Grieve, Rick, and Adrienne Helmick. "The influence of men's self-objectification on the drive for muscularity: Self-esteem, body satisfaction and muscle dysmorphia." *International Journal of Men's Health* 7.3 (2008): 288.
21 Freeman, Samuel. "Illiberal libertarians: Why libertarianism is not a liberal view." *Philosophy & Public Affairs* 30.2 (2001): 105–151.
22 Rorty, Richard. "Universality and truth." In Robert B. Brandom (ed.), *Rorty and his critics*. Blackwell, 2000: 1–30.
23 Miller, Joshua D., et al. "Vulnerable narcissism is (mostly) a disorder of neuroticism." *Journal of Personality* 86.2 (2018): 186–199.
24 Bruni, Luigino, and John Milbank. "Martin Luther and the different spirits of capitalism in Europe." *International Review of Economics* 66 (2019): 221–231.
25 Iyer, Ravi, et al. "Understanding libertarian morality: The psychological roots of an individualist ideology." PLoS One 7.8 (2010): e42366.
26 Forti, Simona. *Totalitarianism: a borderline idea in political philosophy*. Stanford University Press, 2024.
27 Tomšič, Samo. "The antisociality of capitalism (some preliminary reflections)." In Ben Gook (ed.), *Libidinal economies of crisis times: The psychic life of contemporary capitalism*. Transcript, 2024: 89.
28 Poldrugo, F. "Anxiety disorders and addictions." *European Psychiatry* 11.S4 (1996): 155s.

29 Freud, Sigmund. *The ego and the id.* Simon and Schuster, 2019.
30 Freud, Sigmund. *Inhibitions, symptoms and anxiety.* Norton, 1977.
31 Samuels, Robert. "(Liberal) narcissism." In Yannis Stavrakakis (ed.), *Routledge handbook of psychoanalytic political theory.* Routledge, 2019: 151–161.
32 Casey, Edward S. "Freud's theory of reality: a critical account." *The Review of Metaphysics* (1972): 659–690.
33 Samuels, Robert. *The psychopathology of political ideologies.* Routledge, 2021.
34 Freud, Sigmund. *Group psychology and the analysis of the ego.* Hogarth Press, 1949.
35 Samuels, Robert. "Beyond Hillary Clinton: Obsessional narcissism and the failure of the liberal class." In Robert Samuels, *Psychoanalyzing the Left and Right after Donald Trump: Conservatism, liberalism, and neoliberal populisms.* Springer, 2016: 31–59.
36 Needles, William. "The pleasure principle, the constancy principle, and the primary autonomous ego." *Journal of the American Psychoanalytic Association* 17.3 (1969): 808–825.
37 Freud, Sigmund. *Dora: An analysis of a case of hysteria.* Simon and Schuster, 1997.
38 Samuels, Robert. "Pathos, hysteria, and the Left." In Robert Samuels, *Žižek and the rhetorical unconscious: Global politics, philosophy, and subjectivity.* Springer, 2020: 7–31.
39 Schierup, Carl-Ulrik, and Stephen Castles. "Migration, minorities and welfare states." *Migration in the Global Political Economy* 17 (2011): 15–40.
40 Foster, Roger. "Social character: Erich Fromm and the ideological glue of neoliberalism." *Critical Horizons* 18.1 (2017): 1–18.
41 Smith, Robert C. *Society and social pathology: A framework for progress.* Palgrave Macmillan, 2017.
42 Pettman, Ralph. *Psychopathology and world politics.* World Scientific, 2012.
43 Freud, Sigmund. *Moses and monotheism.* Sanzani Edizioni, 2023.
44 Lee, Lester C. *An investigation of Erich Fromm's theory of authoritarianism.* Claremont Graduate University, 1963.
45 de Courville Nicol, Valérie. *Anxiety in middle-class America: Sociology of emotional insecurity in late modernity.* Routledge, 2021.
46 Seligman, Adam B. "Individualism as principle: Its emergence, institutionalization, and contradictions." *Indiana Law Journal* 72 (1996): 503.
47 Samuels, Robert. "(Liberal) narcissism." In Yannis Stavrakakis (ed.), *Routledge handbook of psychoanalytic political theory.* Routledge, 2019: 151–161.
48 Samuels, Robert. *Political pathologies from* The Sopranos *to* Succession*: Prestige TV and the contradictions of the "liberal" class.* Routledge, 2023.
49 Samuels, Robert. *Political pathologies from* The Sopranos *to* Succession*: Prestige TV and the contradictions of the "liberal" class.* Routledge, 2023.
50 Freud, Sigmund. *Three case histories.* Simon and Schuster, 2008.
51 Lukes, Steven. *Individualism.* ECPr Press, 2024.
52 Pasewark, Kyle. "Predestination as a condition of freedom." *Lutheran Quarterly* 12 (1998): 57–78.
53 Layton, Richard A. "Martin Luther and John Calvin on predestination." *Essays in History* 26 (1982).
54 Freud, Sigmund. *Civilization and its discontents.* Broadview Press, 2015.
55 Lasch, Christopher. "The culture of narcissism." In Rupert Wilkinson (ed.), *American social character.* Routledge, 2019: 241–267.
56 Ross, Nathaniel. "The 'as if' concept." *Journal of the American Psychoanalytic Association* 15.1 (1967): 59–82.

57 Forsyth, James J. Biblical faith and Erich Fromm's theory of personality. Dissertation, University of Ottawa, 1968.
58 Burms, Arnold. "Individual autonomy and a culture of narcissism." *Ethical Perspectives* 5.4 (1998): 277–284.
59 Freud, Sigmund. *Civilization and its discontents.* Broadview Press, 2015.

Chapter 7

The Freudian Theory of Ideology

In *Totem and Taboo*, we learn about how particular ideologies are shaped by specific psychopathologies on a cultural and individual basis.[1] Starting with his theory of the primary processes, we discover why and how social order is developed, maintained, and internalized. In fact, the surprising aspect of Freud's notion of the super-ego is that it is essentially a psychotic agency that feeds a traditional ideology.[2] Moreover, Freud attaches this internal mental agency to the first period of culture (animism), which is then transcended by religion and finally science.[3] As we shall see by referring to *Group Psychology and the Analysis of the Ego*, a key defining aspect of the transition from traditional animistic society to authoritarian religion is the centralization of power around a single idealized object.[4]

Freud's Basic Historical Model

A key passage from *Totem and Taboo* introduces Freud's basic historical model that he will utilize throughout his work:

> Writers maintain that in the course of time three such systems of thought, three great world systems came into being: the animistic (mythological), the religious, and the scientific. Of these animism, the first system is perhaps the most consistent and the most exhaustive, and the one which explains the nature of the world in its entirety. This first world system, of mankind is now a psychological theory. It would go beyond our scope to show how much of it can still be demonstrated in the life of to-day, either as a worthless survival in the form of superstition, or in living form, as the foundation of our language, our belief, and our philosophy.
>
> (*TT*: 2019)

Freud's perspective on ideology is thus shaped by his endorsement of the theory that human civilization has moved through three major belief systems: animism, religion, and science.[5] Moreover, as we shall see, Freud also relates diverse cultural systems to particular psychopathologies:

DOI: 10.4324/9781003773948-7

> In one way the neuroses show a striking and far-reaching correspondence with the great social productions of art, religion and philosophy, while again they seem like distortions of them. We may say that hysteria is a caricature of an artistic creation, a compulsion neurosis, a caricature of a religion, and a paranoic delusion, a caricature of a philosophic system. In the last analysis this deviation goes back to the fact that the neuroses are asocial formations; they seek to accomplish by private means what arose in society through collective labour.
>
> (*TT*: 2015–2016)

The important move in this passage is to tie three different social activities to specific psychopathologies: The end result is that we have to see culture and individual subjectivity as shaping each other in an ongoing dialectic.[6]

At the foundation of Freud's theory is the argument that there is a fundamental conflict between sex and society:

> In analyzing the impulse of the neuroses one learns that motive powers of sexual origin exercise the determining influence in them, while the corresponding cultural creations rest upon social impulses and on such as have issued from the combination of egotistical and sexual components. It seems that the sexual need is not capable of uniting men in the same way as the demands of self-preservation; sexual satisfaction is in the first place the private concern of the individual.
>
> (*TT*: 2016)

A central idea here is that humans are driven by sexual desire, but this drive is anti-social and also does not enhance self-preservation; rather, sexual desire caters to the isolated individual and resists the possibility of uniting humans.[7] In other words, sex is represented as the foundation of a libertarian ideology dedicated to the unregulated impulses of the borderline, anti-social individual.[8]

It is vital to stress that Freud has an expanded notion of sexuality, which includes all of our basic impulses.[9] In fact, in the case of neurosis, he posits that sexual desire is inherently anti-social:

> Genetically the asocial nature of the neurosis springs from its original tendency to flee from a dissatisfying reality to a more pleasurable world of phantasy. This real world which neurotics shun is dominated by the society of human beings and by the institutions created by them; the estrangement from reality is at the same time a withdrawal from human companionship.
>
> (*TT*: 2016)

From this radical perspective, Freud helps us to see how the libertarian ideology of the Right is based on fantasy, desire, and the resistance to social regulation.[10] In other words, the promotion of liberty and the individual pursuit of happiness results in a loss of social regulation and collective unity.

If the Right is driven by the pleasure principle, Freud posits that modern science and psychoanalysis are driven by overcoming both the pursuit of pleasure and the psychology of omnipotent thinking:

> Animism, the first conception of the world which man succeeded in evolving, was therefore psychological. It did not yet require any science to establish it, for science sets in only after we have realized that we do not know the world and that we must therefore seek means of getting to know it. But animism was natural and self-evident to primitive man; he knew how the things of the world were constituted, and as man conceived himself to be. We are therefore prepared to find that primitive man transferred the structural relations of his own psyche to the outer world, and on the other hand we may make the attempt to transfer back into the human soul what animism teaches about the nature of things.
>
> (*TT*: 2107)

Freud's argument here is that the initial form of social organization (animism) was based on humans treating their own thoughts as being natural and determined by the pure perception of reality, but with science, the key move is to realize that we do not know things, and therefore we have to find a way to discover the truth of reality.[11] He adds that by taking on a scientific perspective concerning internal reality, we can transfer what animistic cultures say about nature back onto our understanding of how the human mind works.

Animism, Traditionalism, and Paranoid Knowledge

The first way that Freud seeks to explain traditional ideology and culture is to argue that in animistic societies, the origin and the meaning of many of their social practices remains unknown to the people who perform them:

> The taboo prohibitions lack all justification and are of unknown origin. Though incomprehensible to us they are taken as a matter of course by those who are under their dominance. Wundt calls taboo the oldest unwritten code of law of humanity. It is generally assumed that taboo is older than the gods and goes back to the pre-religious age.
>
> (*TT*: 1954–1955)

According to this theory, which is shared by many structuralist anthropologists, cultural traditions and practices do not rely on meaning or conscious knowledge since they can by practiced without knowing their origins or significance.[12] In other words, if we want to study traditional ideologies, it makes no sense to ask people why they believe what they believe or practice what they practice since this form of social order is not based on meaning or conscious awareness.[13]

Freud's conception of traditional ideology, then, challenges most other theories of ideology since it is no longer a question of inner belief or conscious thinking. In his development of the theory of the human conscience (the super-ego), Freud makes the radical claim that our internalized morality is not intentional: "Originally the punishment for the violation of a taboo was probably left to an inner, automatic arrangement. The violated taboo avenged itself" (*TT*: 1956). By saying that the punishment for a violation of social norms and laws is automatic, Freud is not saying that is it biological or natural; instead, his theory of traditional ideology relies on the notion that people do not fully control their own minds, and much of the content of their thinking has been the result of the internalization of cultural content through imitation, but they still think that these ideas are the products of their own thinking.[14]

Most other theories of ideology fail to grasp this foundational principle, which concerns the way people use the primary processes to both project and introject cultural morality. From Freud's perspective, the essence of traditional ideology is centered on the internalization of an unintentional moral system:

> We may say, however, that we deal with a series of restrictions which these primitive races impose upon themselves; this and that is forbidden without any apparent reason; nor does it occur to them to question this matter, for they subject themselves to these restrictions as a matter of course and are convinced that any transgression will be punished automatically in the most severe manner. There are reliable reports that innocent transgressions of such prohibitions have actually been punished automatically. For instance, the innocent offender who had eaten from a forbidden animal became deeply depressed, expected his death and then actually died.
>
> (*TT*: 1957–1958)

I prefer to call this form of culture and subjectivity, traditional instead of primitive in order to reduce the stigmatization and to insist that all human thought and culture is originally based on this type of internalized, automatic morality: As Freud articulates with his theory of the primary processes, our thinking is fundamentally unintentional, irrational, and indirect.[15]

In contrast to Aristotle's attempt to rationalize the traditional social order by seeing it as inevitable, natural, and intentional, Freud bases this form of ideology on the confusion among socially constructed values, internalized representations, and perceptions of the external world. From this Freudian perspective, conspiracy theories are not rare mental events; instead, our default way of processing information and relating to others is through the identification with a social order based on symbolic connections:

> Something like a theory seems to underlie all these prohibitions, it seems as if these prohibitions are necessary because some persons and objects possess a dangerous power which is transmitted by contact with the object so charged, almost like a contagion. The quantity of this dangerous property is also taken into consideration. Some persons or things have more of it than others and the danger is precisely in accordance with the charge. The most peculiar part of it is that anyone who has violated such a prohibition assumes the nature of the forbidden object as if he had absorbed the whole dangerous charge.
>
> (*TT*: 1958)

Not only do people identify in a non-conscious way with the symbolic social order that surrounds them: They also treat others in relation to this mythical and mystical form of social understanding.[16] As Freud insists, all societies have to create stability and order by regulating sex and violence, and this desire for social order often relies on magical thinking and the fear of the contagious spread of evil.[17]

This notion that humans are afraid of the spread of a dangerous power can be equated with the conservative phobic ideology.[18] Since people replace real risks with symbolic substitutes, they seek protection from potentially threatening people and objects.[19] Moreover, in response to the anxiety generated by the perceived threat, individuals and societies provide mechanisms for avoidance and protection. In this structure, the conservative desire for protection is enhanced by the social provision of order established through the repetition of symbolic rituals.[20]

Freud adds that on the level of primary processes and animistic cultures, the sacred and the profane are often treated as if they were the same thing: "The prohibition derived from this attribute is also designated as taboo, and lastly taboo, in the literal sense, includes everything that is sacred, above the ordinary, and at the same time dangerous, unclean and mysterious" (*TT*: 1959). By uniting the sacred and the dangerous together, Freud highlights how what we experience as good and evil is derived from a purely symbolic interpretation that has little connection to reality.[21]

One of the major moves by Freud here is to tie our conscience to a set of primitive mechanisms, and here we see why the super-ego is irrational, unintentional, and indirect: "the moral and customary prohibitions which we ourselves obey may have some essential relation to this primitive taboo the explanation of which may in the end throw light upon the dark origin of our own 'categorical imperative'" (*TT*: 1959). In other words, our conscience is a primitive mechanism derived from the power of symbolic and social thoughts to make causal connections where they do not actually exist in nature or reality.[22]

The primary processes also do not follow the law of non-contradiction since the same objects are considered to be both loved and hated:

> The main characteristic of the psychic constellation which has thus gone under fixation lies in what one might call the ambivalent behaviour of the individual to the object, or rather to an action regarding it. The individual constantly wants to carry out this action (the act of touching), he sees in it the highest pleasure, but he may not carry it out, and he even abominates it. The opposition between these two streams cannot be easily adjusted because—there is no other way to express it—they are so localized in the psychic life that they cannot meet. The prohibition becomes fully conscious, while the surviving pleasure of touching remains unconscious, the person knowing nothing about it. If this psychological factor did not exist the ambivalence could neither maintain itself so long nor lead to such subsequent manifestations.
>
> (*TT*: 1967)

From Freud's perspective, there is a fundamental ambivalence shaping human desire since we love what we hate and are repulsed by what we desire.[23] However, this ambivalence can itself by interpreted as stemming from the fundamental conflict between social morality and human drives: What we desire is often what society prohibits, and what society prohibits is what we desire.[24] Moreover, this ambivalence is repressed into the unconscious as the two opposing sources are separated and maintained in different psychological locations. One of the goals then of analytic treatment is to provide a space for this ambivalence to emerge and be clarified.

The Ideology of Center-Left Narcissism

In drawing a parallel between the organization of traditional society and the formation of the unconscious in the individual, Freud seeks to bring together social analysis and depth psychology:

> The transferability and reproductive power of the prohibition reflect a process which harmonizes with the unconscious pleasure and is very much facilitated through the psychological determinants of the unconscious. The pleasure of the impulse constantly undergoes displacement in order to escape the blocking which it encounters and seeks to acquire surrogates for the forbidden in the form of substitutive objects and actions. For the same reason the prohibition also wanders and spreads to the new aims of the proscribed impulse. Every new advance of the repressed libido is answered by the prohibition with a new severity. The mutual inhibition of these two contending forces creates a need for

> discharge and for lessening the existing tension, in which we may recognize the motivation for the compulsive acts.
>
> (*TT*: 1967)

In making this connection between obsessive-compulsive neurosis and the mentality of animistic cultures, Freud emphasizes that in both, we are dealing with the conflict between prohibition and desire, yet the way that obsessional neurotics try to overcome this conflict is not only by displacing the object of their desire but also engaging in compulsive rituals.[25]

In the case of obsessional-compulsive neurosis, we find that the purifying rituals represent an attempt to combine together the original impulse with a reaction against it:

> In the neurosis there are distinctly acts of compromise which on the one hand may be regarded as proofs of remorse and efforts to expiate and similar actions; but on the other hand they are at the same time substitutive actions which recompense the impulse for what has been forbidden. It is a law of neurotic diseases that these obsessive acts serve the impulse more and more and come nearer and nearer to the original and forbidden act.
>
> (*TT*: 1967–1968)

While it may appear that Freud's main point here is that there are no real differences between neurotics and animistic cultures, we shall see that while neurotics use repression as their main defense mechanism, animistic cultures rely on the psychotic process of projection.[26]

From an ideological perspective, we can equate the obsessive-compulsive neurosis with the narcissistic personality since the desire to see oneself as good is actualized by having others admire one's ideal ego.[27] Thus, in what we now call virtue signaling, one attempts to have one's morality and competence admired by others in order to convince oneself that one is good and pure.[28] This process entails separating morality from the underlying desires it is seeking to regulate and contain: Through the process of repression, antisocial drives are hidden from the self in order to maintain a sense of being morally good and innocent.[29]

It is important to point out that one of the problems with Freud's theory at this point is that he tends to confuse the primary processes and the unconscious:

> First of all it must be said that it is useless to question savages as to the real motivation of their prohibitions or as to the genesis of taboo. According to our assumption they must be incapable of telling us anything about it since this motivation is "unconscious" to them. But following the model of the compulsive prohibition we shall construct the history of taboo as follows: Taboos are very ancient prohibitions which at one time were forced upon a generation of primitive people from without, that is, they probably were

> forcibly impressed upon them by an earlier generation. These prohibitions concerned actions for which there existed a strong desire.
>
> (*TT*: 1968–1969)

While the unconscious is caused by repression and the desire to maintain a certain idealized self-image in the structure of center-Left narcissism, the non-conscious ideology of traditional ideology is based on the way that internal thoughts are treated as if they were perceptions of the external world; meanwhile external cultural content is introjected, yet one is not aware that their thoughts are being derived from an outside source.[30]

As Freud demonstrates, one reason why external ideology can be transmitted without conscious awareness is that it is maintained through unexamined traditions:

> The prohibitions maintained themselves from generation to generation, perhaps only as the result of a tradition set up by paternal and social authority. But in later generations they have perhaps already become "organized" as a piece of inherited psychic property. Whether there are such "innate ideas" or whether these have brought about the fixation of the taboo by themselves or by co-operating with education no one could decide in the particular case in question.
>
> (*TT*: 1969)

The radical move here is to posit that ideologies can shape societies and individuals without anyone understanding where they come from or what purpose they actually serve.[31] Since they may be circulated through imitation and identification, they do not require conscious awareness, and this lack of awareness poses a problem for most theories of ideology.

The Roots of Conservative Ideology

The power of imitation also relates to the fear that conservatives have of contagious social transgressions:

> An individual who has violated a taboo becomes himself taboo because he has the dangerous property of tempting others to follow his example. He arouses envy; why should he be allowed to do what is prohibited to others? He is therefore really contagious, in so far as every example incites to imitation and therefore he himself must be avoided.
>
> (*TT*: 1970)

Since conservatives believe that any transgression of social morality will lead others to do the same, they must do anything they can in order to isolate and avoid the person who appears to be dangerous.[32]

The irrationality of this conservative phobic ideology becomes apparent in its use of the primary processes:

> But a person may become permanently or temporarily taboo without having violated any taboos, for the simple reason that he is in a condition which has the property of inciting the forbidden desires of others and of awakening the ambivalent conflict in them. Most of the exceptional positions and conditions have this character and possess this dangerous power. The king or chieftain rouses envy of his prerogatives; everybody would perhaps like to be king. The dead, the newly born, and women when they are incapacitated all act as incitements on account of their peculiar helplessness, while the individual who has just reached sexual maturity tempts through the promise of a new pleasure. Therefore all these persons and all these conditions are taboo, for one must not yield to the temptations which they offer.
>
> (*TT*: 1970–1971)

According to this theory, what produces anxiety and the phobic desire to avoid this feeling is the fear that someone will induce others to transgress the social morality.[33] While in a traditional society, these fears and mechanisms of avoidance are enacted through shared social rituals and moral beliefs, in the case of a neurotic phobia, the conflict is internalized and repressed.[34]

With neurotic anxiety, the main cause for fear is a lack of the ability to predict what will happen next.[35] Since one is confronted with an unknowable event or feeling, one feels vulnerable to a direct harm and a potential loss of life. Of course, this threat can be triggered by something that is not actually life-threatening, like public speaking, but the lack of protection and prediction causes a triggering of the biological flight-or fight-responses where bodily energy is generated in order to respond to a perceive risk.[36] In the case of conservative ideology, the call for protection and the insistence on social law and order is generated in response to social change and the encounter with different types of people.[37]

Freud adds that anxiety and the desire for protection can be triggered by both internal impulses and the fear of losing the social order:

> This danger really exists if we substitute the known impulses for the unconscious desires. It consists in the possibility of imitation, as a result of which society would soon be dissolved. If the others did not punish the violation they would perforce become aware that they want to imitate the evil doer.
>
> (*TT*: 1971)

From the conservative perspective, all threats have to be punished so that society does not fall into anarchy.[38] Moreover, Freud locates in both traditional and conservative ideology, a shared fear of the power of the leader:

> These races consider it necessary to watch over their kings to see that they use their powers in the right way; they are by no means sure of their good intentions or of their conscientiousness. A strain of mistrust is mingled with the motivation of the taboo rules for the king.
>
> (*TT*: 1983)

Since animistic cultures show a profound distrust in regard to the power of their leaders, it becomes necessary to explain why people might move to idealize these authorities and suspend all of their doubts and fears.

Idealization, Transference, and Authoritarian Ideology

In *Group Psychology and the Analysis of the Ego*, Freud sets out to determine the reasons people will submit to the will of others as they suspend their own reality testing and reason. The first processes that he attaches to authoritarian ideology represents a return to his earlier theory of contagious social influences:

> contagion, also intervenes to determine the manifestation in groups of their special characteristics, and at the same time the trend they are to take. Contagion is a phenomenon of which it is easy to establish the presence, but that it is not easy to explain. It must be classed among those phenomena of a hypnotic order, which we shall shortly study. In a group every sentiment and act is contagious, and contagious to such a degree that an individual readily sacrifices his personal interest to the collective …
>
> (*GPAE*: 10)

The concept of the contagion is thus a key to understanding Freud's theory of authoritarian ideology because it helps to explain why individuals would sacrifice their own interests for the group.[39]

By grounding his conception of authoritarianism in his experience with hypnosis, he seeks to account for why people succumb to the suggestions made by the person they have placed in the position of idealized authority:

> We know to-day that by various processes an individual may be brought into such a condition that, having entirely lost his conscious personality, he obeys all the suggestions of the operator who has deprived him of it, and commits acts in utter contradiction with his character and habits. The most careful investigations seem to prove that an individual immersed for some length of time in a group in action soon finds himself—either in consequence of the magnetic influence given out by the group, or from some other cause of which we are ignorant—in a special state, which must resemble the state of "fascination" in which the hypnotized individual finds himself in the hands of the hypnotizer.
>
> (*GPAE*: 11–12)

What Freud draws from this theory is the connection between the individual in the group and the person being hypnotized.[40] Since Freud started out his therapeutic technique by hypnotizing his patients, he has a great deal of knowledge about this topic, yet it also should be mentioned that Freud developed psychoanalysis by breaking away from hypnosis, and so in many ways, the psychoanalytic process is in opposition to suggestion.[41]

Freud posits that the artificial social group functions by effacing the will of the individual subject:

> In order to make a correct judgement upon the morals of groups, one must take into consideration the fact that when individuals come together in a group all their individual inhibitions fall away and all the cruel, brutal and destructive instincts, which lie dormant in individuals as relics of a primitive epoch, are stirred up to find free gratification. But under the influence of suggestion groups are also capable of high achievements in the shape of abnegation, unselfishness, and devotion to an ideal.
>
> (*GPAE*: 17)

In this approach to suggestion and contagious behavior, Freud sees these processes as having both positive and negative effects; thus, suggestion can allow us to escape our own narcissism to accomplish important social goals, yet it also can function to free us to express our inhibited destructive impulses.[42]

While authoritarians tend to remove inhibitions, they also can produce a lack of reality testing:

> And, finally, groups have never thirsted after truth. They demand illusions, and cannot do without them. They constantly give what is unreal precedence over what is real; they are almost as strongly influenced by what is untrue as by what is true.
>
> (*GPAE*: 19–20)

It is this lack of distinction between truth and fiction that most disturbs Freud about the authoritarian personality.[43] Furthermore, what helps to trigger this type of unreason is the way that people submit uncritically to the suggestions of the idealized leader:

> Moreover, he ascribes both to the ideas and to the leaders a mysterious and irresistible power, which he calls 'prestige'. Prestige is a sort of domination exercised over us by an individual, a work or an idea. It entirely paralyses our critical faculty, and fills us with astonishment and respect. It would seem to arouse a feeling like that of fascination in hypnosis.
>
> (*GPAE*: 21)

In the same way that the hypnotized person will do whatever the hypnotist tells them to do, an authoritarian personality will follow the commands of the idealized leader without question.[44]

This submission to a higher power is coupled by Freud with the emotional feedback effect between members of the group:

> The individual loses his power of criticism, and lets himself slip into the same emotion. But in so doing he increases the excitement of the other people, who had produced this effect upon him, and thus the emotional charge of the individuals becomes intensified by mutual interaction.
> (*GPAE*: 28)

When the individual regresses to the primitive state of consciousness in front of the powerful leader, this suspension of reality testing through immersion is shared by other people who submit to the same power.[45] There are thus two processes occurring here: individuals are subjected to the will of the leader, and the followers imitate each other's regressive thinking.[46] Freud reveals here the key to authoritarian ideology since it relies on the suspension of reality testing and the release of uninhibited drives through the submission to an idealized leader or idea.

Authoritarian figures then gain control by getting their followers to regress to the level of the helpless child in front of the all-powerful caregiver, and this regression to infantile helplessness is coupled with a sense of empowerment:

> This mechanism for the intensification of emotion is favoured by some other influences which emanate from groups. A group impresses the individual with a sense of unlimited power and of insurmountable peril. For the moment it replaces the whole of human society, which is the wielder of authority, whose punishments the individual fears, and for whose sake he has submitted to so many inhibitions. It is clearly perilous for him to put himself in opposition to it, and it will be safer to follow the example of those around him and perhaps even "hunt with the pack". In obedience to the new authority he may put his former "conscience" out of action, and so surrender to the attraction of the increased pleasure that is certainly obtained from the removal of inhibitions.
> (*GPAE*: 28)

Freud explains here why people may join a cult or political movement since he connects subjective submission to the removal of inhibitions and the illusion of unlimited power in the face of extreme dangers.[47] Taking advantage of the combination of the primary processes coupled with the relational desire for salvation, leaders are able to influence our minds by turning our subjection into a source of perceived power and freedom.

As a type of shock doctrine, Freud posits that what often draws people to powerful leaders and ideologies is the panic and anxiety caused by the loss of social bonds:

> A hint to the same effect, that the essence of a group lies in the libidinal ties existing in it, is also to be found in the phenomenon of panic, which is best studied in military groups. A panic arises if a group of that kind becomes disintegrated. Its characteristics are that none of the orders given by superiors are any longer listened to, and that each individual is only solicitous on his own account ...
>
> (*GPAE*: 45)

For Freud, the example of a social panic reveals that the group has always been constituted by a "primitive" need for social order.[48] He adds that the organizing principle can also be the shared hatred of another group:

> The leader or the leading idea might also, so to speak, be negative; hatred against a particular person or institution might operate in just the same unifying way, and might call up the same kind of emotional ties as positive attachment.
>
> (*GPAE*: 53)

It is interesting that for Freud, a leader or an idea can play the role of organizer, and so on the level of social psychology, there is no real difference between people and ideas.[49] As Lacan insists, our social reality is structured by signifiers, and so the social bond is based on the linking of symbolic representations.[50] From this perspective, we are never really dealing with other people since we only know them as a collection of social signs. Moreover, since each signifier is defined in opposition to other signifiers, self-identity relies on being opposed to other people, and here we see why hatred can be such a powerful organizing principle: Due to the fact that the group has to define itself in opposition to other groups, internal group identity often relies on the conservative phobic hatred of the out-group.[51]

Freud stresses that within the structure of the authoritarian relationship, we often find the spread of emotions through a process of identification:

> There is a third particularly frequent and important case of symptom formation, in which the identification leaves any object relation to the person who is being copied entirely out of account. Supposing, for instance, that one of the girls in a boarding school has had a letter from someone with whom she is secretly in love which arouses her jealousy, and that she reacts to it with a fit of hysterics; then some of her friends who know about it will contract the fit, as we say, by means of mental infection. The mechanism is that of identification based upon the

> possibility or desire of putting oneself in the same situation. The other girls would like to have a secret love affair too, and under the influence of a sense of guilt they also accept the pain involved in it. It would be wrong to suppose that they take on the symptom out of sympathy. On the contrary, the sympathy only arises out of the identification ...
>
> (*GPAE*: 64)

Through the development of an authoritarian mindset, the subjects in the group all express the same emotional reaction because they all identify with the same sense of suffering. In other words, in this context, empathy does not lead to social progress; instead, it results in a regressive form of identification:[52]

> We already begin to divine that the mutual tie between members of a group is in the nature of an identification of this kind, based upon an important emotional common quality; and we may suspect that this common quality lies in the nature of the tie with the leader. Another suspicion may tell us that we are far from having exhausted the problem of identification, and that we are faced by the process which psychology calls "empathy [Einfühlung]" and which plays the largest part in our understanding of what is inherently foreign to our ego in other people.
>
> (*GPAE*: 66)

Freud's radical gesture is to base our empathic understanding of others on an unconscious identification, and from this perspective, our initial comprehension of others relies on imitating their emotional responses.[53]

Not only does Freud compare the submission to the authoritarian leader to the process of hypnosis, but he also draws a parallel between this ideology and the state of passionate love:

> The tendencies whose trend is towards directly sexual satisfaction may now be pushed back entirely, as regularly happens, for instance, with the young man's sentimental passion; the ego becomes more and more unassuming and modest, and the object more and more sublime and precious, until at last it gets possession of the entire self-love of the ego, whose self-sacrifice thus follows as a natural consequence. The object has, so to speak, consumed the ego. Traits of humility, of the limitation of narcissism, and of self-injury occur in every case of being in love; in the extreme case they are only intensified, and as a result of the withdrawal of the sensual claims they remain in solitary supremacy.
>
> (*GPAE*: 74–75)

The sublime object of love is thus derived in part from the destruction of the lover's ego, which is demanded by the idealization of the beloved: The self-sacrificing lover becomes full of humility because the ego has been transcended by the ego ideal.[54]

What is so interesting is that Freud once again equates the love of the other to an idea as he describes how the devotion to a love object matches the commitment to a social ideal:

> Contemporaneously with this "devotion" of the ego to the object, which is no longer to be distinguished from a sublimated devotion to an abstract idea, the functions allotted to the ego ideal entirely cease to operate. The criticism exercised by that faculty is silent; everything that the object does and asks for is right and blameless. Conscience has no application to anything that is done for the sake of the object; in the blindness of love remorselessness is carried to the pitch of crime. The whole situation can be completely summarised in a formula: The object has taken the place of the ego ideal.
>
> (*GPAE*: 75)

The sublime object of authoritarian ideology is here generated from the substitution of the object for the conscience, and so the lover is not only deaf and dumb but also amoral.[55] As a theory of the freely chosen submission of the subject to an idealized Other, this theory of love reveals that the more we devote ourselves to the ideals of others, the more we eliminate our ability to make moral and epistemological judgments.[56]

As Freud insists, the model of the organized social group is the hypnotic relationship because the group requires our complete submission:

> From being in love to hypnosis is evidently only a short step. The respects in which the two agree are obvious. There is the same humble subjection, the same compliance, the same absence of criticism, towards the hypnotist just as towards the loved object. There is the same absorption of one's own initiative; no one can doubt that the hypnotist has stepped into the place of the ego ideal.
>
> (*GPAE*: 77)

This replacement of the ego ideal with the object in hypnosis, love, and authoritarian ideology means that the biggest risk idealization poses is that it has the power to make individuals suspend all criticism as they become immersed in a singular object of attention.[57] In fact, Freud emphasizes that hypnosis is made possible by a form of deep focus:

> The hypnotist is the sole object, and no attention is paid to any but him. The fact that the ego experiences in a dream-like way whatever he may request or assert reminds us that we omitted to mention among the functions of the ego ideal the business of testing the reality of things.
>
> (*GPAE*: 77)

It is thus the focus on the singular object that effaces the subject and removes reality testing and moral judgment.[58]

For Freud, when multiple people replace their ego ideals with the same object, a fanatical group is formed, and like any type of cult, this group loses its ability to employ the reality principle or a moral conscience:

> Some of its features—the weakness of intellectual ability, the lack of emotional restraint, the incapacity for moderation and delay, the inclination to exceed every limit in the expression of emotion and to work it off completely in the form of action—these and similar features, which we find so impressively described in Le Bon, show an unmistakable picture of a regression of mental activity to an earlier stage such as we are not surprised to find among savages or children.
>
> (*GPAE*: 81–82)

Freud's theory of group regression helps us to comprehend why people submit to destructive leaders and follow irrational conspiracy theories.[59]

Freud's pessimistic conclusion is that the due to way we become absorbed in the ideas and ideals of an idealized Other, we are prone to fanaticism, racism, and other destructive attitudes:

> We thus have an impression of a state in which an individual's separate emotion and personal intellectual act are too weak to come to anything by themselves and are absolutely obliged to wait till they are reinforced through being repeated in a similar way in the other members of the group. We are reminded of how many of these phenomena of dependence are part of the normal constitution of human society, of how little originality and personal courage are to be found in it, of how much every individual is ruled by those attitudes of the group mind which exhibit themselves in such forms as racial characteristics, class prejudices, public opinion, etc.
>
> (*GPAE*: 82)

By stressing the dependency and prejudice of the authoritarian group, Freud demonstrates why individuals may submit to a destructive leader. Moreover, this theory helps us to understand the link between racism, sexism, homophobia, and authoritarian ideology.[60]

The Authoritarian Structure of the Church and Army

As Freud develops his theory of authoritarian ideology, he relates this structure to the foundations of religions and armies:

> A church and an army are artificial groups, that is, a certain external force is employed to prevent them from disintegrating and to check

> alterations in their structure. As a rule a person is not consulted or is given no choice, as to whether he wants to enter such a group; any attempt at leaving it is usually met with persecution or with severe punishment, or has quite definite conditions attached to it.
>
> (*GPAE*: 42)

Here Freud stresses that authoritarian groups often rely on force and threats of violence in order to maintain cohesion; in other words, it is not simply a process of idealization that accounts for the solidarity of the collective organization; rather, members know that anyone who attempts to leave will be punished and harmed.[61]

Although Freud clearly believes that the authoritarian group is maintained through the threat of violence, he also highlights the important role love plays:

> In a church (and we may with advantage take the Catholic Church as a type) as well as in an army, however different the two may be in other respects, the same illusion holds good of there being a head—in the Catholic Church Christ, in an army its Commander-in-Chief—who loves all the individuals in the group with an equal love. Everything depends upon this illusion; if it were to be dropped, then both Church and army would dissolve, so far as the external force permitted them to. This equal love was expressly enunciated by Christ: "Inasmuch as ye have done it unto one of the least of these my brethren, ye have done it unto me." He stands to the individual members of the group of believers in the relation of a kind elder brother; he is their father surrogate.
>
> (*GPAE*: 42–43)

Freud posits here that for a church or army to be sustained, the members must not only be afraid of leaving or criticizing the leader, they must also feel that they are all loved equally by the head of the institution.[62] As a benevolent father-figure, the leader must treat all of the members with the same underlying care.

Although, Freud relates the maintenance of the authoritarian group to the combination of love and fear, he sees the lack of freedom of the individual as the key ingredient:

> It would appear as though we were on the right road towards an explanation of the principal phenomenon of Group Psychology—the individual's lack of freedom in a group. If each individual is bound in two directions by such an intense emotional tie, we shall find no difficulty in attributing to that circumstance the alteration and limitation which have been observed in his personality.
>
> (*GPAE*: 45)

From this perspective, there should be a clear opposition between authoritarian and libertarian ideologies, yet what we often find today is that these opposing belief systems are brought together through the establishment of coalitions where people freely submit to an idealized leader who promises salvation.[63]

As Freud had previously indicated, one way that this type of coalition is built and maintained is by rallying around a shared hated other.[64] Freud also stated above that the authoritarian leader can allow individuals to access their impulses without inhibition.[65] However, even if the leader does appear to love the followers, anyone outside the group must be a target of hate:

> Therefore a religion, even if it calls itself the religion of love, must be hard and unloving to those who do not belong to it. Fundamentally indeed every religion is in this same way a religion of love for all those whom it embraces; while cruelty and intolerance towards those who do not belong to it are natural to every religion.
>
> (*GPAE*: 50–51)

This cruelty towards outsiders is thus a key aspect of all authoritarian groups and ideologies.[66] In fact, Freud argues that it does not matter if the social group is a church, army, or political ideology since what determines the structure is the underlying authoritarian relationship:

> If another group tie takes the place of the religious one—and the socialistic tie seems to be succeeding in doing so—, then there will be the same intolerance towards outsiders as in the age of the Wars of Religion; and if differences between scientific opinions could ever attain a similar significance for groups, the same result would again be repeated with this new motivation.
>
> (*GPAE*: 51)

As we find with non-religious cults, the content of the group belief system is less important than the combination of idealization, submission, and fear.[67]

In the next chapter, I develop this relationship between authoritarian ideology and religion by providing a close reading of Freud's *Moses and Monotheism*. As the term mono-theism indicates, a key to the transition from traditional animism to authoritarian religion is the focus on the One person who knows or cares. Thus, as Lacan argues in relation to transference, we love the person we put in the position of the Subject Supposed to Know.[68]

Notes

1 Freud, Sigmund. "Totem and taboo." In Sigmund Freud, *Collected works*. Vol. 9. Delphi Classics, 2017. Hereafter cited as "*TT*" in this chapter.

2 Traetta, Luigi, and Federica Doronzo. "Super-ego after Freud: A lesson not to be forgotten." *Elementa: Intersections between Philosophy, Epistemology and Empirical Perspectives* 1.1–2 (2022): 153–161.
3 Rice, Emanuel. "Freud, religion, and science." *Journal of the American Academy of Psychoanalysis* 27.3 (1999): 397–406.
4 Freud, Sigmund. *Group psychology and the analysis of the ego.* Hogarth Press, 1949. Hereafter cited as "*GPAE*" in this chapter.
5 Barre, Weston La. "Freudian biology, magic, and religion." *Journal of the American Psychoanalytic Association* 26.4 (1978): 813–830.
6 Samuels, Robert. *The psychopathology of political ideologies.* Routledge, 2021.
7 Freud, Sigmund. *Civilization and its discontents.* Broadview Press, 2015.
8 Whynacht, Ardath J. "Citizens of nowhere": Diffractive engagements with borderline personality disorder. Dissertation, Concordia University, 2017.
9 Freud, Sigmund. *Three essays on the theory of sexuality: The 1905 edition.* Verso Books, 2017.
10 Samuels, Robert. *Žižek and the rhetorical unconscious: Global politics, philosophy, and subjectivity.* Springer, 2020.
11 Moser, Franz. "Beyond Sigmund Freud's *Totem and Taboo* vision for the future—the omnipotence of thought." *International Journal of Foresight and Innovation Policy* 13.3–4 (2018): 187–194.
12 Lévi-Strauss, Claude. *Structural anthropology.* Basic books, 2008.
13 Rossi, Ino. "The unconscious in the anthropology of Claude Lévi-Strauss 1." *American Anthropologist* 75.1 (1973): 20–48.
14 Knight, Robert P. "Introjection, projection and identification." *The Psychoanalytic Quarterly* 9.3 (1940): 334–341.
15 Freud, Sigmund. *Psychopathology of everyday life.* W. W. Norton & Company, 1966.
16 Kroeber, Alfred Louis. "*Totem and Taboo*: an ethnologic psychoanalysis." *American Anthropologist* 22.1 (1920): 48–55.
17 Brottman, Mikita. "Psychoanalysis and magic: Then and now." *American Imago* 66.4 (2009): 471–489.
18 Helminen, Vilja, Marko Elovainio, and Markus Jokela. "Clinical symptoms of anxiety disorders as predictors of political attitudes: A prospective cohort study." *International Journal of Psychology* 57.2 (2022): 181–189.
19 Freud, Sigmund. "Analysis of a phobia in a five-year-old boy." In Sigmund Freud, *Collected papers.* Vol. 3 Basic Books, 1955: 149–289.
20 Hatemi, Peter K., and Rose McDermott. "Dispositional fear and political attitudes." *Human Nature* 31.4 (2020): 387–405.
21 DiCenso, James J. "*Totem and Taboo* and the constitutive function of symbolic forms." *Journal of the American Academy of Religion* 64.3 (1996): 557–574.
22 Weiss, Edoardo. "Regression and projection in the super-ego." *The International Journal of Psycho-analysis* 13 (1932): 449.
23 Kris, Anton O. "The conflicts of ambivalence." *The Psychoanalytic Study of the Child* 39.1 (1984): 213–234.
24 Graubert, David N., and Joseph S. A. Miller. "On ambivalence." *The Psychiatric Quarterly* 31 (1957): 458–464.
25 Graubert, David N., and Joseph S. A. Miller. "On ambivalence." *The Psychiatric Quarterly* 31 (1957): 458–464.
26 Hurry, Anne, Jack Novick, and Kerry Kelly Novick. "Freud's concept of projection." *Journal of Child Psychotherapy* 4.2 (1976): 75–88.
27 Lacan, Jacques. "Remarque sur le rapport de Daniel Lagache." In Jacques Lacan, *Écrits.* Éditions du Seuil, 1966: 647–684.

28 Samuels, Robert. "(Liberal) narcissism." In Yannis Stavrakakis (ed.), *Routledge handbook of psychoanalytic political theory*. Routledge, 2019: 151–161.
29 Samuels, Robert. "Beyond Hillary Clinton: obsessional narcissism and the failure of the liberal class." In Robert Samuels, *Psychoanalyzing the Left and Right after Donald Trump: Conservatism, liberalism, and neoliberal populisms*. Springer, 2016: 31–59.
30 Freeman, Thomas. "Aspects of defence in neurosis and psychosis." *The International Journal of Psycho-Analysis* 40 (1959): 199.
31 Dalal, Farhad. "The social unconscious and ideology: In clinical theory and practice." In Earl Hopper and Haim Weinberg (eds.), *The social unconscious in persons, groups and societies*. Routledge, 2018: 243–263.
32 Robson, David. "The threat of contagion can twist our psychological responses to ordinary interactions, leading us to behave in unexpected ways." Retrieved from www.counsellingresources.co.nz/uploads/3/9/8/5/3985535/fear_of_coronavirus_is_changing_our_psychology.pdf (accessed March 25, 2026).
33 Perini, Mario. "Panic and pandemics: From fear of contagion to contagion of fear." In Halina Brunning (ed.), *Psychoanalytic reflections on a changing world*. Routledge, 2018: 213–232.
34 Park, Anna, Nicole Sharp, and William Ickes. "Social anxiety is contagious." In Theresa M. Robinson (ed.), *Social anxiety: Symptoms, causes and techniques*. Nova Science, 2009: 79–91.
35 Lacan, Jacques. *Anxiety: The seminar of Jacques Lacan, book X*. Polity Press, 2011.
36 Kunimatsu, Melissa M., and Monica A. Marsee. "Examining the presence of anxiety in aggressive individuals: The illuminating role of fight-or-flight mechanisms." *Child and Youth Care Forum* 41 (2012).
37 Wenzelburger, Georg. "Parties, institutions and the politics of law and order: How political institutions and partisan ideologies shape law-and-order spending in twenty western industrialized countries." *British Journal of Political Science* 45.3 (2015): 663–687.
38 West, Robin. "Law, rights, and other totemic illusions: Legal liberalism and Freud's theory of the rule of law." *University of Pennsylvania Law Review* 134 (1985): 817.
39 Murphy, James. "On the authoritarian personality." In Beverley Best, Werner Bonefeld, and Chris O'Kane, *The Sage handbook of Frankfurt School critical theory*. Vol. 2. Sage, 2018: 899–915.
40 Adorno, Theodor W. "Freudian theory and the pattern of fascist propaganda." In Andrew Arato and Hike Gebhardt (eds.), *The essential Frankfurt school reader*. Basil Blackwell, 1951: 118–137.
41 Freud, Sigmund. "The dynamics of transference." In James Strachey (ed.), *The standard edition of the complete psychological works of Sigmund Freud*. Vol. 12. Hogarth Press, 1953–1974: 97–108.
42 Koritar, Endre. "The leader's hypnotic influence and the creation of alternate reality." *The American Journal of Psychoanalysis* 82.3 (2022): 349–363.
43 Hassan, Steven A., and Alan W. Scheflin. "Understanding the dark side of hypnosis as a form of undue influence exerted in authoritarian cults and online contexts: Implications for practice, policy, and education." In Julie H. Linden, Giuseppe De Benedittis, Laurence I. Sugarman, and Katalin Varga (eds.), *The Routledge international handbook of clinical hypnosis*. Routledge, 2024: 755–772.
44 Katchen, Martin H. "Brainwashing, hypnosis, and the cults." *Australian Journal of Clinical and Experimental Hypnosis* 20 (1992): 79–79.
45 Meissner, William W. "Notes on identification I: Origins in Freud." *The Psychoanalytic Quarterly* 39.4 (1970): 563–589.

46 Rudnytsky, Peter L. "Freud, Ferenczi, Fromm: The authoritarian character as magic helper." *Fromm Forum* 18 (2015): 5–10.
47 Spitz, Renée A., and Hella Freud Bernays. "The genesis of magical and transcendent cults." *American Imago* 29.1 (1972): 2–10.
48 Dupuy, Jean-Pierre. "Panic and the paradoxes of the social order." In Wolfgang Palaver and Petra Steinmair-Pösel (eds.), *Passions in economy, politics, and the media: in discussion with Christian theology.* LIT Verlag Münster, 2005: 215–233.
49 Hinshelwood, Robert D. "Ideology and identity: A psychoanalytic investigation of a social phenomenon." *Psychoanalysis, Culture & Society* 14 (2009): 131–148.
50 Miller, Jacques-Alain, Paul Verhaeghe, and Ellie Ragland. *Jacques Lacan and the other side of psychoanalysis: Reflections on Seminar XVII.* Vol. 6. Duke University Press, 2006.
51 Rasoulikolamaki, Sahar, Surinderpal Kaur, Alena Zhdanava, and Noor Aqsa Nabila Mat Isa. "In-group and out-group identity construction in extremist discourse: a critical multimodal approach." *Behavioral Sciences of Terrorism and Political Aggression* 17.4 (2025): 377–395.
52 Bloom, Paul. *Against empathy: The case for rational compassion.* Random House, 2017.
53 Pigman, George W. "Freud and the history of empathy." *The International Journal of Psycho-analysis* 76.2 (1995): 237.
54 González-Torres, Miguel Ángel, and Aranzazu Fernandez-Rivas. "Desire and submission." In Margarita Sáenz-Herrero (ed.), *Psychopathology in women: Incorporating gender perspective into descriptive psychopathology.* Springer, 2019: 377–389.
55 Žižek, Slavoj. *The sublime object of ideology.* Verso, 1989.
56 Benjamin, Jessica. *The bonds of love: Psychoanalysis, feminism, and the problem of domination.* Pantheon, 2013.
57 Samuels, Robert. "Victim politics: Psychoanalyzing the neoliberal conservative counter-revolution." In Robert Samuels, *Psychoanalyzing the Left and Right after Donald Trump: Conservatism, liberalism, and neoliberal populisms.* Springer, 2016: 7–29.
58 Bachner-Melman, Rachel, and Pesach Lichtenberg. "Freud's relevance to hypnosis: A reevaluation." *American Journal of Clinical Hypnosis* 44.1 (2001): 37–50.
59 Samuels, Robert. "Freud's contagion." In Robert Samuels, *Viral rhetoric: Psychoanalysis, philosophy, and politics after Covid-19.* Springer International Publishing, 2021: 61–77.
60 Haider, Asad. "Authoritarianism and ideology." *CLCWeb: Comparative Literature and Culture* 23.1 (2021): 2.
61 Cheliotis, Leonidas K. "Violence and narcissism: A Frommian perspective on destructiveness under authoritarianism." *Canadian Journal of Sociology* 36.4 (2011): 337–360.
62 Eizirik, Cláudio Laks. "Freud's group psychology, psychoanalysis, and culture." In Ethel Spector Person (ed.), *On Freud's "Group psychology and the analysis of the ego".* Routledge, 2018: 155–173.
63 Wood Jr, James E. "Religious fundamentalism and the New Right." *Journal of Church and State* 22 (1980): 409.
64 Vella, Norman. "Freud on groups." In Chris Oakley (ed.), *What is a group?: A New Look at Theory in Practice.* Routledge, 2019: 8–38.
65 Anzieu, Didier. "Freud's group psychology: Background, significance, and influence." In Ethel Spector Person (ed.), *On Freud's "Group psychology and the analysis of the ego".* Routledge, 2018: 39–60.
66 Frankel, Jay. "The narcissistic dynamics of submission: The attraction of the powerless to authoritarian leaders." *American Journal of Psychoanalysis* 82.3 (2022): 384.

67 Kenny, Dianna T. *God, Freud and religion: The origins of faith, fear and fundamentalism.* Routledge, 2015.
68 Diatkine, Gilbert. "Lacan and the transference." *The International Journal of Psychoanalysis* 104.4 (2023): 722–736.

Chapter 8

Freud, Religion, and Identity Politics

The Formation of Global Subjectivity and Ideology

In the previous chapter, I outlined Freud's theories of traditional, conservative, and authoritarian ideologies. One of my main arguments is that psychoanalysis provides the most effective way of understanding how ideology functions in the world today because it places these belief systems in a dialectic between social organization and individual psychopathology.[1] As we shall see in this chapter, a close analysis of his *Moses and Monotheism* can further helps us to comprehend religion, the roots of authoritarian ideology, and the problematic nature of identity politics.[2] Moreover, this comprehension of distinct ideologies will lead us to a new theory of globalism as both an integrated psychological model and a way to promote global progress and global subjectivity.[3]

Freud's Liberal Method

Written during the time of the rise of the National Socialists in Germany, Freud's *Moses and Monotheism* can be read today as an effective critique of both authoritarian ideology and contemporary Left-wing identity politics.[4] Even though Freud knew that his "race" was under attack, and he was forced to go into exile, he still insisted on producing a text that de-idealizes his own identity group.[5] Ultimately, what this misunderstood book demonstrates is the need to affirm ambivalence and ambiguity as the foundations of our cultural relationships; instead of trying to idealize the history and leaders of the Jewish people, Freud locates a primary doubling in relation to Moses.[6] In an act of intellectual bravery, he splits Moses into two different people: An Egyptian Moses and a Jewish one. This splitting places at the heart of the Jewish tradition a divided subject, and this division reflects how every identity is ambivalent and ambiguous.[7]

At the start of his book, Freud states that he is aware that he is undermining the idealization of Moses by the Jewish people, yet he argues that no consideration of "national interests" will push him to set aside the truth (*MM*: 3).[8] As an Enlightenment rationalist and liberal ideologue, the founder of psychoanalysis affirms a commitment to both reason and universalism; in

DOI: 10.4324/9781003773948-8

other words, he separates psychoanalytic practice and theory from a defense of specific national and religious identities and idealization.[9] From this perspective, we can affirm that at the heart of psychoanalysis, one finds a calling into question of all cultural identities and investments as a mode of global subjectivity is affirmed.[10] In fact, the very act of Freud writing this book during the time that it was composed represents a desire for truth and a rejection of religious and ethnic identity within a global context.

One of Freud's main sociological claims, borrowed from Otto Rank, is that almost every nation builds up its identity through the production of myths that glorify a national hero (*MM*: 7).[11] Thus, the idealization of the great individual leads to the idealization of the nation, and in the case of Moses, the Jewish people sought to idealize themselves by repressing the true history of Moses himself.[12] Therefore, by de-idealizing Moses, Freud is also de-idealizing his own "race." Freud adds that the original source for this idealizing tendency revolves around the child's idealization of the father (*MM*: 9).[13] From his perspective, the idealization of nations relies on the idealization of leaders, and the idealization of leaders is derived from the idealization of the father: It is this mode of idealization that we can ascribe to authoritarian ideology.[14]

In combining individual psychology with cultural history, Freud shows why psychoanalysis does not privilege the individual over society or society over the individual; there is an inherent dialectic between individual development and cultural history, and so it is unfair to attack psychoanalysis for only caring about the isolated individual.[15] Moreover, Freud affirms that the original idealization of the parents by the child is followed by a critical attitude towards the father, and so the basic relation to the parent and the nation is one of ambivalence since two opposing perspectives are always at play (*MM*: 10).[16]

The Divided Subject

The doubled relation to parents and the nation is reflected in the idea that there were two different people named Moses: one is a Jew from a humble family, and the other is an Egyptian from a royal family.[17] However, in an act of audacity, Freud claims that the Jewish Moses is actually a fictious one; in other words, the great Jewish leader did not exist, and he was created in order to hide the true origins of this mythologized national hero (*MM*: 13).[18] By claiming that this essential Jew is not really a Jew, Freud places the other in the heart of Jewish identity.[19]

Freud uses the example of the doubled Moses to not only call into question all idealized nationalism and identity but also to define the foundations of monotheism.[20] Since the real Moses was Egyptian, he practiced a polytheistic religion, and so the question is how did the Jewish people become committed to a "unique, omnipotent, unapproachable" singular God?[21]

While the Egyptians believed in many local gods with magical powers, the Jews replaced this traditional spirituality and ideology with "sublime abstraction" (*MM*: 17). Moreover, in contrast to the Egyptian belief in life after death, the Jews gave up on immortality.[22]

Freud attempts to explain the transition to monotheism by arguing that the Egyptian Moses was a king who attempted to consolidate his power by imposing a new monotheistic belief system (*MM*: 21). Acting as a vanishing mediator, the Egyptian Moses, then, serves as a transition from primitive animism to religious monotheism.[23] This transitional figure also reveals how religion is often used to consolidate political power.[24] Since this leader wanted to be the only one that people would listen to and obey, he promoted a religion based on a singular higher power. We see here how to this day, religion is often a political tool connected to nationalism and authoritarian ideology.[25]

In tracing the linguistic connections among the Egyptian sun god Aton and the Hebrew word for lord, Adonai, Freud posits that the buried truth of Moses can be found in the "primeval unity" of language (*MM*: 27).[26] Thus, very little of the Jewish tradition is original since it is derived from re-written sources. Of course, this theory of cultural history echoes Freud's understanding of how the primary processes in individual minds rely on the rewriting of the past often through linguistic substitutions, associations, and displacements.[27]

De-idealizing History

One aspects of Freud's de-idealization of Jewish mythology can be found in his analysis of the ritual of circumcision: While some believe that it was the Jewish tradition that introduced this practice, Freud relates that it was already performed for a long time in Egypt (*MM*: 29).[28] In order to defend this point, Freud adds a footnote where he declares that it may look like his is using history in an arbitrary, self-serving manner, but in reality, it is religious history that is shaped by motivated distortions, and he intends to discover the repressed truth determined by secret motives (*MM*: 30 n.1).[29] The over-all effect of his method is to reveal how behind every stable identity and identification, we find multiple, conflicting sources and misrepresentations.

It is vital to stress that in the face of the Nazi demonization of the Jews, Freud does not seek to idealize his own people and history; instead, he de-idealizes religion and nationalism in order to provide an unbiased, universal liberal perspective dedicated to discovering the truth of reality.[30] In terms of the Jews claiming that they have been chosen by God as a special people, and this relationship is demonstrated through the ritual of circumcision, Freud claims that the people who practice this act always feel superior to the "unclean" people who do not follow this proud custom (*MM*: 33).[31] For example, Turks will attack a Christian for being "an uncircumcised dog."[32]

This reference to Shakespeare's *Othello* is intended to show that this "traditional" ritual does not belong only to the Jewish people, and it can be used as a way of putting down people who are not part of the same identity group.[33] As a marker of difference, Freud believes that the Egyptian leader Moses used circumcision as a way of making a new group of people a "holy nation" separate from all of the other cultural groups around them (*MM*: 34).[34] Once again, we see here the shared roots of religion and nationalism: In order for a people to feel superior and different, they have to engage in symbolic acts that separate them from other groups deemed inferior and unholy.[35]

One of Freud's central insights is that every nation and religion relies on re-writing history and texts in order to fit the purposes of the leaders (*MM*: 62).[36] In fact, Freud argues that the only way to approach the truth of a people's past is to examine the contradictions and omissions circulating in their texts (*MM*: 52). Freud goes as far as saying that the distortion of a text is similar to a murder, and while it may be easy to commit the crime, there are always traces left behind.[37] It is then the task of the historian to read past writings in order to determine the truth of what really happened. Here, Freud compares the method of psychoanalysis to that of the historian since in both cases, the goal is to interpret the defensive distortions in order to attain the truth of past reality.[38] On a fundamental level, Freud is driven by the liberal desire for truth as he seeks out verification for his speculations.

Progress and Barbarism

In part three of his text, Freud turns his attention to the period just before 1938, and he posits that Europe was experiencing a strange combination of Enlightenment progress and barbarism.[39] By referring to both the rise of the Nazis and the Soviet Communists, he locates the same contradictory coalescing of modern values and anti-modern tendencies.[40] Thus, in relation to the Soviet Union, he applauds the elimination of religion and the liberation of sexuality, but he critiques "the most cruel coercion" robbing people of the "freedom of thought" (*MM*: 67).[41] Freud therefore accurately points to the way that the great effort to create a more equal and just society turned into its opposite. He adds that the Germans and Italians also experienced a similar regression to prehistoric barbarism, and only the Catholic Church provided any resistance (*MM*: 67).[42] Yet, he still posits that the Church is the "implacable enemy of all freedom of thought" (*MM*: 67). For Freud, it is thus the freedom to think, which is the most important liberal value to protect: Similar to his use of free association in analytic practice, Freud privileges free thought as the ultimate liberal democratic ideal to protect against the return to barbarism, nationalism, and religion.[43]

As a mode of the return of the repressed, the regression back to an earlier stage of civilization relates to Freud's fundamental belief that old desires, thoughts, and memories can never be fully erased (*MM*: 84).[44] Just as infantile impulses can return in the present, societies that have progressed beyond pure violence and control can always return to their original state.[45] This dialectical theory entails that we should never take freedom or progress for granted since "prehistoric" impulses are always ready to re-surface.[46] Freud adds that between an initial historical event and its return, there is a period of latency or repression where the initial state has been forgotten.[47] According to this theory, a key aspect to the return of past barbarism is the forgetting of the past, which paves the wave for national and religious idealization.

The Primal Horde Revisited

To further illustrate his concept of the return of the past prehistoric period of barbarism, Freud goes back to his analysis of Darwin's theory of the primal horde (*MM*: 102).[48] His main point is that in this initial form of social organization, small groups were dominated by a single, powerful male. This leader, who was also considered to be a father, ruled with unlimited power in a brutal fashion, and all of the women were considered to be his property.[49] Whether we consider this a myth or the actual reality, the main point is that social organization starts in a violent way as a singular entity has all of the power and access to the objects of desire.[50] Moreover, the original structure of the primal horde can be related to the relational desire of libertarian ideology: In this system, the male father-figure is free to act on his impulses without restriction.[51]

After the establishment of the primal horde, the next stage concerns the way the oppressed brothers banded together in order to take power by killing and consuming the primal father-leader (*MM*: 103).[52] Freud uses this myth/history in order to reveal the universality of the Oedipus complex since the brothers who desired to kill the father were driven in part by their desire to access the women he controlled.[53] However, after this act of murder and cannibalism is enacted, the brothers feel guilt for their actions, and so they decide to create a social order built around the regulation of sex and violence (*MM*: 104).[54] Through the development of morality and the internalization of the super-ego, a traditional ideology was created that functioned to regulate the drives of the brothers and the father.[55]

Instead of reading Freud's story of prehistoric civilization as a recounting of a historical reality, it is more effective to see that he is using the past in order to define the development of the present.[56] Thus, his effort to explain the return to barbarism in modern Europe relies on his theory of what barbarism means and how it can be overcome both on an individual and collective manner. Unlike evolutionary psychologists, Freud sees the original state of social organization as centered on the dominance of unrestrained males.[57] From this perspective, the rise of fascism in Europe represents both a return to the primal horde of male dominance and the submissive idealization of this powerful figure.[58] In other terms, fascism combines together the libertarian impulses of the masculine drive with the authoritarian desire for salvation.

As we see in the current rise of masculine Right-wing leaders, their power is made possible by the fact that they can get other people to support their dominance, and one way that this support is generated is through the ideology of the center-Right.[59] Since traditional morality reinforces the social hierarchy, it can serve as a way to naturalize and rationalize male dominance. Also, the conservative need to focus on an enemy of social order helps to protect the masculine leader and reinforces the desire for strict law and order.[60] Fascism, then, represents the bringing together of the extreme version of four different ideologies: libertarian, authoritarian, conservative, and center-Right.

In the context of current geopolitics, we can use Freud's theory to see how Putin's attack on Ukraine represents a return to masculine barbarism and a rejection of the union of brothers who have renounced violence and the hording of resources.[61] Institutions, then, like the European Union embody a liberal social contract based on guilt and shared renunciation; however, in order for this new social union to be achieved, it is first necessary to kill off the primal violent father-leader.[62] From this perspective, Left-wing postmodern social movements are founded on reversing the primal order of masculine barbarism and the traditional morality structure in order to break the master's monopoly on violence and resources, and yet this needed violent revolution has to also be renounced once the master has been removed.[63]

We learn from Freud's model that at the foundations of social order, we find violence and the idealization of this violence.[64] Moreover, Freud ties this history to a gendered narrative where it is men and fathers who represent the essence of barbarism, yet the ultimate liberal goal is to constitute a universal union transcending gender and violence.[65] Since morality and law require an act of instinctual renunciation, it is vital to place at the center of modern democracy the need to delay sexual and violent impulses. Freud is therefore not a libertarian who seeks to endorse the liberation of the drives; instead, he affirms the need to acknowledge the tension between drives and society.

After Idealization and Identity Politics

Freud is clearly at his most audacious and speculative here, but there is a method to his madness: Behind every identity and identification, he locates ambivalence and self-division.[66] The other is always inside of the self, and a dialectic shapes history and individual development.[67] Thus, against the current culture of polarization and splitting, he locates a twisted foundation where opposites affect each other. In this structure, every identity becomes problematized, and every effort at idealization becomes de-idealized.[68] We, thus, never fully escape our barbarism on a collective or individual level, and the only hope is to find better ways to delay our gratification by investing in shared social institutions, yet these institutions cannot be dependent on repressing the truth or stopping critical thinking and reality testing.[69]

One would think that at a time when Jews were constantly being threatened based on their identity, Freud would seek to defend their heritage and support his own race, but instead, he sought to call into question the traditions and beliefs of the Jewish people.[70] Refusing to engage in idealization and identification, Freud presents an early critique of identity politics.[71] In fact, his representation of his own Jewish identity is coupled with a criticism of what he sees as particular Jewish traits. For instance, he claims that Jews tend to have a high opinion of themselves and that this arrogance keeps them separate from other groups, which often leads to them being hated by others (*MM*: 134).[72] This Jewish mode of national and racial narcissism is related to the belief that they are really the chosen people of the idealized father-God (*MM*: 134).[73] Here, we see that in the structure of national narcissism, the ideal ego is recognized by the ego ideal.

In the case of Jewish tradition and belief, Freud sees Moses as the idealized master who helps to provide a single cause to the complex question of how this group was able to become so unified.[74] Employing the "great man of history" theory, the Jewish people have repressed the divided and complicated nature of Moses and his followers so that they could idealize the past and their own identities (*MM*: 136).[75] Freud adds that people have a strong need for an authority who they can admire and to whom they can submit (*MM*: 140).[76] Here, transference is tied to the authoritarian personality, which helps to explain why people suspend their own interests and reality testing in order to subject themselves to an idealized master.[77] Due to an infantile desire for a strong protective father, there is a common fantasy of being saved and protected by a hero (*MM*: 140).[78] In all of these idealized masters, Freud finds the same combination of decisive thought, strength of will, forcefulness of deeds, and self-reliance (*MM*: 140).[79] In other words, the submissive subjects need a sociopathic leader who must be trusted even when he acts in a ruthless manner.

While Freud's focus on the father and masculine traits may appear to be a sexist idealization of men, his main point it to show how this type of gender identification is highly destructive.[80] It is the violence of the borderline father who is then idealized by the submissive masses who seek to find protection from loss and harm.[81] Idealization and violence then are linked together as Freud uses his theory of the doubled Moses to combine together the law and paternal violence.[82] Since the Jews believed in a God who was unique, omnipotent, and eternal, they established an idealized father who was prone to lay down incomprehensible, irrational demands (*MM*: 140).[83] Moreover, the Jewish prohibition against making a representation of God subordinated sense perception to an abstract idea (*MM*: 144).[84] In fact, Freud sees in this restriction an instinctual renunciation coupled with an investment in pure spirituality. In this triumph of culture over sensation, the Jewish people were able to produce certain intellectual skills, and yet this commitment to a spiritual ideal left them prone to abuse and hatred (*MM*: 147).[85]

Due to the fact that the Jews favored ideas over perceptions, they also privileged the father over the mother since there are visible signs of maternity, but the role of the father is a mental supposition (*MM*: 150).[86] Likewise, since God is invisible, the investment in him relies on privileging thought over perception.[87] From this perspective, the development of religion relies on a substitution of sensation with thought. Freud adds that the narcissism of the religious person may be heightened by a sense that they have mastered their own impulses by submitting to a higher order of belief (*MM*: 150).[88] Yet, at the heart of Freud's analysis of religion is the notion that it is the leaders who decide what is sacred, and these father-figures determine what is morally good and bad in order to protect their own self-interest.[89] In other words, morality is determined by the desire of the powerful to protect their privilege (*MM*: 156).[90] Furthermore, when subjects idealize these leaders and their morality, they are buying into a system that can only oppress them. In this context, Freud understands circumcision as a mode of castration and punishment that signals a submission to the father's violent will (*MM*: 156).[91]

Freud adds that people, like himself, who have no belief in a higher power must feel envious towards those who do not have to question anything because God provides an answer to every inquiry (*MM*: 157).[92] As a liberal Enlightenment thinker, Freud exclaims that religious belief overwhelms reason and science, and so it is his task to determine where this type of idealization comes from. On one level, Freud traces the foundations of belief back to the infantile desire for protection against a dangerous world, but he also argues that what really drives belief is the satisfaction of our wishes and illusions that meet truth half-way (*MM*: 166).[93] From this perspective, there really was a great leader who unified a people; however, this leader was really a series of people who were neither divine nor ideal. In fact, Freud traces masculine power and privilege to the willingness to exploit and use other people coupled with the idealization of leaders and fathers by the people who are being used.[94]

Mixed with idealization, Freud highlights how feelings of guilt often function to help people endure hard times and misfortune (*MM*: 172). Since no one can live up to all of the religious laws and prohibitions, they feel that they only have themselves to blame when things go wrong.[95] So even if the chosen people constantly have to deal with oppression and abuse, they turn blame inward as they continue to idealize a higher power: The flip-side of the idealization of the father-God is thus internalized self-hatred (*MM*: 173).[96] Moreover, God's severity is rationalized by the need to be punished for sinful thoughts and feelings. In this masochistic dynamic, the more severe the prohibitions and punishments coming from God tend to be, the more people feel they are being treated justly due to their inability to follow impossible moral demands.[97] For Freud, the repressed memory of the original murder of the primal father triggers a mode of guilt that is insatiable, but we do not have to believe in this primal inheritance since it is clear that most religions control their adherents through the generation of guilt internalized in the super-ego.[98] Freud adds that the stricter the religious dictates become, the more people harbor a secret hostility towards God, which only adds to their guilt and desire for punishment.

Psychoanalytic Politics and Ethics

In reading *Moses and Monotheism*, we discover that we can never escape the threat of a return to pre-modern barbarism.[99] We also learn that psychoanalysis offers a critical perspective on identity, identification, idealization, nationalism, and religion. Although some therapists and analysts would like to transform treatment into a form of identity affirmation or empathic identification, it should be clear that Freud locates an essential ambivalence and ambiguity at the heart of every identity.[100] Freud also makes the curious claim that the best way for Jewish people to defend their race is to be open and honest about the past; part of this process relies on giving up the idealization of the self and the Other.

As we see in the current conflict in Israel, when a people idealize their nation and religion, they no longer are committed to reason and the reality principle.[101] Some people argue that a time of crisis is no time to take on a critical perspective, yet as Freud's own text reveals, it is precisely during the aftermath of a trauma that people have to repress their immediate drives for revenge and self-pity. For Freud, the ultimate value remains the freedom to think, and it is this freedom that is often threatened by war, nationalism, and religion.

Freud argues that deeply buried in the Jewish tradition, one finds the foundations of the modern liberal desire for justice and truth:

> To one part of the people the Egyptian Moses had given another and more spiritual conception of God, a single God who embraces the whole world, one as all-loving as he was all-powerful, who, averse to all ceremonial and magic, set humanity as its highest aim a life of truth and justice.
>
> (*MM*: 61)

Thus, according to this theory, underlying the desire for salvation through the idealization of a higher power, we also find a buried liberal call for truth and justice through the imposition of a universal belief system.[102]

The question then for globalism is how can one get people to invest in an ideology dedicated to universality, justice, and truth without turning to some form of religious idealization or traditional spirituality.[103] Moreover, if we want to move beyond the narcissism of nationalism so that we can embrace a global mode of governance and social order, how do we avoid the pitfalls of the conservative fear of the other and libertarian call for unlimited freedom? [104] In other words, how do we both recognize and balance the distinct relational desires that shape the major ideologies and psychopathologies?

As we saw in our discussion of Steven Pinker's articulation of global progress, the key to global progress and consciousness must relate to the dominance of modern science and democratic law, yet, we have also found that the Enlightenment call to move beyond all previous belief systems has never been achieved, and one reason for this failure may be that we cannot simply wish away the underlying relational desires shaping specific ideologies and psychopathologies. For instance, during and after the COVID pandemic, it was clear that it was not effective to simply tell people the science behind vaccines or the need for a shared, collective response; rather, it was also necessary to get people to trust the government and to ignore misleading conspiracy theories.[105] Furthermore, much of the resistance to the governmental response to the virus was fueled by a libertarian desire for individual freedom.[106] The question, then is should we simply ignore all of the competing ideologies, or is there some way of combining them together in an effective manner?

It is my argument that an integrated theory of globalism has to recognize the need to learn how to separate, moderate, and relate the eight major ideologies shaping our world since each of these belief systems represent an extreme form of a foundational relational desire. Since people desire order, salvation, liberation, accommodation, protection, admiration, equality, and the truth, we have to find a way to cater to the non-extreme versions of these demands.[107] In fact, every effective mode of communication does have to rely on some level of trust and belief as one seeks to represent the truth for both individuals and groups.[108] The trick is how do we reduce ideological conflict by privileging the less extreme version of each of the ideologies.

Ideologies and Psychological Agencies

As Freud's work indicates, the first stage of this process is to clearly understand the human desires underlying each belief system. Next, we need to learn how to respond to these desires but not fuel the extreme and rigid forms that they demand. As Freud articulates in his book on Moses, one way of approaching this need for an integrated theory of globalism is to examine the differences and relations among distinct psychological agencies.[109] Freud begins his analysis of the specific mental regions in the following manner:

> Now we distinguish from our mental life-which we see to be an apparatus consisting of several hierarchies, districts, or provinces-one region,

> which we term the "real Ego," from another which we call the "Id." The Id is the older; the Ego has developed out of it through the influence of the outer world as the bark develops around a tree.
>
> (*MM*: 122)

While Freud wants to present the different mental provinces that shape the human mind, he is quick to add that these locations do not relate to specific brain regions: "I will add here that the topography of the psyche I have here developed has in general nothing to do with cerebral anatomy" (*MM*: 123). Thus, even though Freud started as a neurologist, he makes a clear break here from basing the organization of the mind on the structure of the brain.[110]

Unfortunately, while Freud does reject anatomical localization in *Moses and Monotheism*, he tends to fall back on a false belief in the notion of inherited, prehistoric mental content.[111] Thus, in order to further clarify the different mental agencies and how they relate to specific ideologies, it is necessary to examine his *The Ego and the Id* where he endeavors to clearly distinguish discrete forms of the ego.[112] Even though many people who know Freud's theory think that there are only three mental agencies, the id, ego, and super-ego, we shall see how in reality, he develops seven different ones: the id, the ego, the super-ego, the reality-ego, the pleasure-ego, the ideal ego, and the ego ideal.[113] While Freud himself does not always keep these distinct agencies separate, my argument is that the dominance of each of these agencies in a culture and an individual lead to a particular ideology and psychopathology.

Freud's first major distinction is to argue that while the id is driven by the pursuit of the pleasure principle, the ego is shaped by reason and the reality principle:

> It is easy to see that the ego is that part of the id which has been modified by the direct influence of the external world through the medium of the Pcpt.-Cs. [perception-consciousness]; in a sense it is an extension of the surface-differentiation. Moreover, the ego seeks to bring the influence of the external world to bear upon the id and its tendencies, and endeavours to substitute the reality principle for the pleasure principle which reigns unrestrictedly in the id. For the ego, perception plays the part which in the id falls to instinct. The ego represents what may be called reason and common sense, in contrast to the id, which contains the passions. All this falls into line with popular distinctions which we are all familiar with; at the same time, however, it is only to be regarded as holding good on the average or "ideally."
>
> (*EI*: 25)

From Freud's perspective, the ego "ideally" attempts to apply reason by substituting the pleasure principle of the id with the reality principle.[114] This liberal ideology stems from the idealization of the desire for truth and the requisite need to delay gratification and circumvent the desire to be liberated from mental tension.[115]

At times, Freud will call this form of the ego, the reality-ego, and he at first connects this mental agency to the perception of external reality:

> By virtue of its relation to the perceptual system it gives mental processes an order in time and submits them to "reality-testing". By interposing the processes of thinking, it secures a postponement of motor discharges and controls the access to motility. This last power is, to be sure, a question more of form than of fact; in the matter of action the ego's position is like that of a constitutional monarch, without whose sanction no law can be passed but who hesitates long before imposing his veto on any measure put forward by Parliament.
>
> (*EI*: 55)

Freud's main argument here is that in order for the mind to test the reality of its perceptions, it has to use thinking to delay movement.[116] In fact, through the use of a metaphor borrowed from politics, Freud represents the reality-ego as having a type of veto power over the rest of the mind.

However, we soon discover that the ego is a very weak master because it has a difficult time controlling and stopping the different, competing mental agencies:

From the other point of view, however, we see this same ego as a poor creature owing service to three masters and consequently menaced by three dangers: from the external world, from the libido of the id, and from the severity of the super-ego. Three kinds of anxiety correspond to these three dangers, since anxiety is the expression of a retreat from danger. As a frontier-creature, the ego tries to mediate between the world and the id, to make the id pliable to the world and, by means of its muscular activity, to make the world fall in with the wishes of the id.

(*EI*: 56)

In this important passage, Freud discusses how the ego has to deal with the demands not only of reality but also of the id and the super-ego.[117] As a weak master, this form of the ego, generates anxiety when it feels danger due to the threats caused by reality, internal drives, and the internalized conscience.[118] Since the reality-ego simply uses reason to test reality, we must differentiate between the ego and the reality-ego.

One problem with Freud's own discourse is that he does not always stay consistent in how he distinguishes the different mental agencies. Thus, it is important to make a clear distinction between the ego in relation to the reality-ego; after all, a key aspect of his general model is that the only way the ego can accurately test reality is if it is not beset by anxiety and the regression to the primary processes.[119] From an ideological perspective, we can affirm that the ego dominates in conservative thinking since the goal is to use avoidance and protection in order to escape internal and external threats.[120] In contrast, the reality-ego defines the liberal dedication to science and the search for empirical truth. Moreover, we know from Descartes that the first step in taking on the perspective of liberal modern science is to suspend all prejudice and presumptions as one ideally views reality from a neutral perspective.[121]

This quest for truth is itself undermined internally by the way that the ego is seduced and controlled by its submission to the id:

> In point of fact it behaves like the physician during an analytic treatment: it offers itself, with the attention it pays to the real world, as a libidinal object to the id, and aims at attaching the id's libido to itself. It is not only a helper to the id; it is also a submissive slave who courts his master's love. Whenever possible, it tries to remain on good terms with the id; it clothes the id's Ucs. [unconscious] commands with its Pcs. [preconscious] rationalizations; it pretends that the id is showing obedience to the admonitions of reality, even when in fact it is remaining obstinate and unyielding; it disguises the id's conflicts with reality and, if possible, its conflicts with the super-ego too. In its position midway between the id and reality, it only too often yields to the temptation to become sycophantic, opportunist and lying, like a politician who sees the truth but wants to keep his place in popular favour.
>
> (*EI*: 65)

By seeking to satisfy the id, the ego is represented here as rationalizing the irrational drives as it pretends that the id is following the dictates of reality.[122] In this description of the sycophantic ego, Freud outlines what we find in center-Right ideology.[123] Since the ideal ego wants to be seen as good and ideal, it pretends to be rational and liberal, but in reality, it functions to justify and rationalize the anti-social aspects of the libertarian id.[124] Moreover, the ideal ego is shaped by a mirroring relation with the ego ideal since the traits of the ideal ego are seen as in conformity with cultural ideals, and as we saw with Aristotle, the privileged subjects main attributes are seen as defining these social ideals.

Psychopathologies, Ideologies, and Mental Agencies

Thus, what we often find in center-Right ideology and discourse is a desire to be seen as being liberal and scientific, yet, what is really driving this ideology and psychopathology is an attempt to hide the individual's investment in the pursuit of pleasure and escape.[125] For instance, many political podcasters and YouTubers like to claim that they are just being neutral and factual when they are really driven by a desire for individual profit, pleasure, privilege, and power.[126] In this structure, the subject seeks to get others to admire its ideal ego by pretending to be liberal when it is actually libertarian.[127]

The reason why we can attach the id to libertarian ideology is that the main aspects of this belief system are the combination of unregulated impulses and emotions coupled with a refusal to accept limits and the need to share with others.[128] Guided by the pleasure principle, the drives in the id take on a borderline personality where the main desire is to be liberated from social control and the tension generated from the super-ego and reality.[129] Since Freud defines the pleasure principle by the avoidance or release of mental tension, he directly opposes the id to the ego and the reality-ego.[130]

One of Freud's radical insights is his theory that the main way to overcome the dominance of the id by the ego is through the process of identification: "It may be that this identification is the sole condition under which the id can give up its objects" (*EI*: 29). This notion of identification plays a key role in the establishment of the super-ego and social subjectivity itself since the main problem Freud wants to solve is why and how do people agree to replace their own sexual and aggressive drives with social dictates?[131] The first theory he provides here is that the way that the Oedipus complex is resolved is by the child replacing the desire for the mother with the law of the father through a process of identification.[132] Therefore, instead of the child wanting to satisfy the drives in the id by accessing the maternal object, the child identifies with the father's desire and regulations.[133]

In an act of identifying with the aggressor, we find the roots of the super-ego and the formation of traditional ideology.[134] Since the main function of traditional society is to provide stability by controlling sex and violence, the subject has to desire to identify with the morality and ideals of the social order while renouncing the immediate satisfaction of the drives in the id.[135] The key to this transformation is the internalization of morality through introjection and identification, and Freud presents this process through his theory of the resolution of the Oedipus complex:

> The broad general outcome of the sexual phase dominated by the Oedipus complex may, therefore, be taken to be the forming of a precipitate in the ego, consisting of these two identifications in some way united with each other. This modification of the ego retains its special position; it confronts the other contents of the ego as an ego ideal or super-ego. (*EI*: 34)

While at times Freud fails to clearly distinguish between the ego ideal and the super-ego, he will later argue that the super-ego judges the ego in relation to the ego ideal.[136] In other terms, guilt and shame are generated when the self does not live up to internalized ideals, and so we have to ask again why and how are these ideals introjected so that the subject feels that the external values are actually internal thoughts?[137]

One of Freud's surprising theories regarding the super-ego is to posit that the conscience does not only represent the internalization of the social regulation of desire, but it also serves to continue the influence the id:

> The super-ego is, however, not simply a residue of the earliest object choices of the id; it also represents an energetic reaction-formation against those choices. Its relation to the ego is not exhausted by the precept: "You ought to be like this (like your father)." It also comprises the prohibition: "You may not be like this (like your father)—that is, you may not do all that he does; some things are his prerogative." This double aspect of the ego ideal derives from the fact that the ego ideal had the task of repressing the Oedipus complex; indeed, it is to that revolutionary event that it owes its existence.
>
> (*EI*: 34)

Even though Freud here equates the ego ideal with the resolution of the Oedipus complex, it should be clear that what he is really saying is that the super-ego judges the ego in relation to ego ideals derived from parents and other social influences.[138] Moreover, society not only tells people what they should not desire—it also articulates what they should desire in relation to their social position.[139] Therefore, the child is called to copy some of the desires of the father, yet other desires are only allowed for the privileged social figure.

The gender hierarchy implicit in this focus on the father is indicative of traditional ideology and the naturalization of the social hierarchy.[140] As Freud makes clear, he begins with attaching the super-ego to the influence of paternal figure, but he soon extends this role to other social influences and authorities:

> Clearly the repression of the Oedipus complex was no easy task. The child's parents, and especially his father, were perceived as the obstacle to a realization of his Oedipus wishes; so his infantile ego fortified itself for the carrying out of the repression by erecting this same obstacle within itself. It borrowed strength to do this, so to speak, from the father, and this loan was an extraordinarily momentous act. The superego retains the character of the father, while the more powerful the Oedipus complex was and the more rapidly it succumbed to repression (under the influence of authority, religious teaching, schooling and reading).
>
> (*EI*: 34)

Since Freud is quick to extend the role of authority in traditional ideology beyond the father, it is essential to see how a diverse set of social influences shape the ideals that the super-ego uses to judge the ego.[141]

As a key aspect of Freud's social theory, the introjection of the super-ego represents the internalization of cultural morality for each subject:

> So long as we had to concern ourselves with the study of what is repressed in mental life, there was no need for us to share in any agitated apprehensions as to the whereabouts of the higher side of man. But now that we have embarked upon the analysis of the ego we can give an answer to all those whose moral sense has been shocked and who have complained that there must surely be a higher nature in man: "Very true," we can say, "and here we have that higher nature, in this ego ideal or super-ego, the representative of our relation to our parents. When we were little children we knew these higher natures, we admired them and feared them; and later we took them into ourselves."
>
> (*EI*: 35)

Here, Freud relates the super-ego to the way children both fear and admire their parents, and there is thus a fundamental ambivalence that is related to our internalization of traditional cultural morality.[142]

Although he is not always consistent on how he differentiates the super-ego from the ego ideal, we know from *Group Psychology and the Analysis of the Ego* that a central distinction between traditional ideology and authoritarian ideology is the way that the focus on a singular object is combined with the submission of the subject who suspends all reality testing.[143] In *The Ego and the Id*, this mode of authoritarian idealization is examined through a discussion of the categorical imperative of the super-ego:

> The super-ego's relation to the later alterations of the ego is roughly similar to that of the primary sexual phase of childhood to later sexual life after puberty. Although it is accessible to all later influences, it nevertheless preserves throughout life the character given to it by its derivation from the father-complex—namely, the capacity to stand apart from the ego and to master it. It is a memorial of the former weakness and dependence of the ego, and the mature ego remains subject to its domination. As the child was once under a compulsion to obey its parents, so the ego submits to the categorical imperative of its super-ego.
>
> (*EI*: 48)

Here the compulsion to obey parental authority is coupled with the compulsive submission of the ego to the super-ego.[144]

What then marks the transition from traditional to authoritarian ideology is the way the super-ego is replaced by a singular object of attention and focus:

> It is easy to show that the ego ideal answers to everything that is expected of the higher nature of man. As a substitute for a longing for the

> father, it contains the germ from which all religions have evolved. The self-judgement which declares that the ego falls short of its ideal produces the religious sense of humility to which the believer appeals in his longing.
>
> (*EI*: 37)

From this perspective, religion uses the super-ego to humble the subject so that the subject turns to the idealized Other for salvation.[145] However, Freud also insists that in this authoritarian structure, the object takes the places of the ego ideal, which is what we find in hypnosis and extreme love.[146]

In *Moses and Monotheism*, Freud adds that in the case of the development of Judaism, we also find a narcissistic component because this group feels that they have been chosen by God for special attention and accommodation.[147] Therefore, instead of the followers of this religion simply effacing their egos and self-esteem, they identify with the idealized Other as their ideal ego is reinforced.[148] However, in distinction to center-Right ideology, here, center-Left narcissism is driven by a desire for admiration coupled with an attempt to repress feelings of guilt, shame, and hostility.[149] This type of repression is explained in *The Ego and the Id* in the following way:

> This double aspect of the ego ideal derives from the fact that the ego ideal had the task of repressing the Oedipus complex; indeed, it is to that revolutionary event that it owes its existence. Clearly the repression of the Oedipus complex was no easy task. The child's parents, and especially his father, were perceived as the obstacle to a realization of his Oedipus wishes; so his infantile ego fortified itself for the carrying out of the repression by erecting this same obstacle within itself. It borrowed strength to do this, so to speak, from the father, and this loan was an extraordinarily momentous act.
>
> (*EI*: 34)

By repressing both the desire for the maternal object and the paternal violent threat against this desire, the narcissistic subject fortifies its ideal ego through a process of identification.[150] In distinction to the internalization of the super-ego, which fills the individual with a sense of guilt and shame, the admiration of the ideal ego by a generalized Other functions to neutralize the super-ego since this Other is placed in a position where all it can do is affirm the externalized idealization of the self.[151]

Freud makes it clear that he sees the ego as the source of repression, and this act of self-deception relies on an internalization of social morality: "we have from the very beginning attributed the function of instigating repression to the moral and aesthetic trends in the ego" (*EI*: 35). From this perspective, the cause of repression and the unconscious is the desire to signal one's conformity to moral standards as one remains invested in anti-social desires.[152] This effort to get the ideal ego admired for its morality can be seen in center-Left virtue-signaling: The main dynamic involves having one's goodness recognized as one continues to act on one's repressed drives.[153]

Even though Freud often ties repression and morality to the super-ego, he clearly indicates here that it is the ideal ego that is the source for repression and hyper-morality.[154] In fact, in a note, he adds the following theory:

> The battle with the obstacle of an unconscious sense of guilt is not made easy for the analyst. Nothing can be done against it directly, and nothing indirectly but the slow procedure of unmasking its unconscious repressed roots, and of thus gradually changing it into a conscious sense of guilt.
>
> (*EI*: 50 n. 1)

While in the case of the traditional super-ego, guilt and morality are conscious, what happens in narcissism is that the guilt itself becomes repressed and unconscious.[155]In other words, one no longer knows that one is being hyper-moral, and in order to protect the ideal ego, guilt has to be hidden from the self.[156] Freud adds that in this structure, "It is possible to discover the repressed impulses which are really at the bottom of the sense of guilt. Thus in this case the superego knew more than the ego about the unconscious id" (*EI*: 53). The idea here is that due to repression, the ego is unaware of the subject's guilt, but the repressed super-ego does know that this guilt is related to repressed drives.[157]

By distinguishing psychotic melancholia from obsessive-compulsive neurosis, Freud is able to show a key difference between the guilt we find in traditional culture and ideology and the guilt we can locate in a narcissistic form of neurosis:

> In melancholia the impression that the super-ego has obtained a hold upon consciousness is even stronger. But here the ego ventures no objection; it admits its guilt and submits to the punishment. We understand the difference. In obsessional neurosis what were in question were objectionable impulses which remained outside the ego, while in melancholia the object to which the superego's wrath applies has been taken into the ego through identification.
>
> (*EI*: 51)

In the case of melancholia, the subject is constantly talking about his or her self-hatred out in the open, yet with the obsessive-compulsive neurosis, self-hatred is repressed and hidden by the idealized ego.[158]

After Freud presents this difference between melancholia and obsessional narcissism, he turns to hysteria as another mode of repression and neurosis:

> The hysterical ego fends off a distressing perception with which the criticisms of its super-ego threaten it, in the same way in which it is in the

> habit of fending off an unendurable object-cathexis—by an act of repression. It is the ego, therefore, that is responsible for the sense of guilt remaining unconscious.
>
> (*EI*: 51–52)

Once again, the ego is seen as the cause of repression and the unconscious: In the effort to defend against distressing thoughts and feelings, the hysteric turns to self-deception.[159] Freud adds that what we really find in hysteria is that the subject attacks the super-ego itself, and in this way, it undermines the master: "We know that as a rule the ego carries out repressions in the service and at the behest of its super-ego; but this is a case in which it has turned the same weapon against its harsh taskmaster" (*EI*: 52). In tying hysteria to an attack on the super-ego and the master, we gain an understanding of how this psychopathology helps to structure Leftist ideology: As the tool of the oppressed, the only way to counter the master's authority is to use the expression of suffering in the call for accommodation.[160]

Although Freud does not say what agency dominates in hysteria, he does indicate that we can connect it to the symptom as a sign of subjective discontent:

> There are certain people who behave in a quite peculiar fashion during the work of analysis. When one speaks hopefully to them or expresses satisfaction with the progress of the treatment, they show signs of discontent and their condition invariably becomes worse. One begins by regarding this as defiance and as an attempt to prove their superiority to the physician, but later one comes to take a deeper and juster view. One becomes convinced, not only that such people cannot endure any praise or appreciation, but that they react inversely to the progress of the treatment. Every partial solution that ought to result, and in other people does result, in an improvement or a temporary suspension of symptoms produces in them for the time being an exacerbation of their illness; they get worse during the treatment instead of getting better. They exhibit what is known as a "negative therapeutic reaction."
>
> (*EI*: 49)

Thus, in opposition to the narcissist who desires praise and admiration, Freud indicates that hysterical subjects cannot tolerate this type of reaction because they are determined to produce a negative reaction.[161] They are therefore invested in their symptom because it serves as a weapon against authority and the super-ego.

As the greatest resistance to analytic treatment, the gain that one gets from suffering in hysteria fuels the negative transference:

> There is no doubt that there is something in these people that sets itself against their recovery, and its approach is dreaded as though it were a

> danger. We are accustomed to say that the need for illness has got the upper hand in them over the desire for recovery. If we analyse this resistance in the usual way—then, even after allowance has been made for an attitude of defiance towards the physician and for fixation to the various forms of gain from illness, the greater part of it is still left over; and this reveals itself as the most powerful of all obstacles to recovery, more powerful than the familiar ones of narcissistic inaccessibility, a negative attitude towards the physician and clinging to the gain from illness.
>
> (*EI*: 49)

Due to what he calls the secondary gain of hysterical suffering, Freud affirms that disempowered people often have to use their victimized status in order to get empathy from others as they form an identity based on their diagnosis.[162]

Since this use of suffering as way of influencing others and stabilizing the identity of the ego is unconscious, it is very hard to know how to counter it.[163] Freud adds that this form of masochism relates to the enjoyment that one can get from punishment: "In the end we come to see that we are dealing with what may be called a 'moral' factor, a sense of guilt, which is finding its satisfaction in the illness and refuses to give up the punishment of suffering" (*EI*: 49).

By enjoying the punishment from the super-ego, the power of the internalized authority is displaced and undermined.[164] Making matters even more complicated is that fact that hysterics do not accept that they are enjoying punishment or that they suffer from unconscious guilt:

> But as far as the patient is concerned this sense of guilt is dumb; it does not tell him he is guilty; he does not feel guilty, he feels ill. This sense of guilt expresses itself only as a resistance to recovery which it is extremely difficult to overcome. It is also particularly difficult to convince the patient that this motive lies behind his continuing to be ill; he holds fast to the more obvious explanation that treatment by analysis is not the right remedy for his case.
>
> (*EI*: 49–50)

From this perspective, the hysterical investment in suffering is the greatest resistance to analysis.[165] Moreover, this theory of hysterical suffering helps us to understand why some people on the Left reject modern science and democracy: Since they are so invested in their suffering as a source of identity and social influence, they do not want to accept the possibility of using reason to replace emotions with objective analysis.[166]

As I will argue in the conclusion of this book, we cannot simply hope that people will take on a global form of consciousness and accept the value of using science and reason to confront and resolve global issues. Instead of simply dismissing the underlying desires and pathologies shaping the eight ideologies, we have to find a way to integrate them by clearly defining them and enabling their less extreme forms.

Notes

1 Samuels, Robert. *The psychopathology of political ideologies.* Routledge, 2021.
2 Freud, Sigmund. *Moses and monotheism.* Sanzani Edizioni, 2023. Hereafter cited as "*MM*" in this chapter.
3 Kayatekin, Serap A., and David F. Ruccio. "Global fragments: Subjectivity and class politics in discourses of globalization." *Economy and Society* 27.1 (1998): 74–96.
4 Chasseguet-Smirgel, Janine. "Some thoughts on Freud's attitude during the Nazi period." In David Meghnagi (ed.), *Freud and Judaism.* Routledge, 2018: 73–92.
5 Watzman, Haim, and Eran J. Rolnik. *Freud in Zion: Psychoanalysis and the making of modern Jewish identity.* Routledge, 2018.
6 Frosh, Stephen. "Freud and Jewish identity." *Theory & Psychology* 18.2 (2008): 167–178.
7 Yerushalmi, Yosef Hayim. *Freud's Moses: Judaism terminable and interminable.* Yale University Press, 1993.
8 Schäfer, Peter. "The triumph of pure spirituality: Sigmund Freud's Moses and Monotheism." *Jewish Studies Quarterly*9.4 (2002): 381–406.
9 Santner, Eric L. "Freud's Moses and the ethics of nomotropic desire." *October* (1999): 3–42.
10 Samuels, Robert. "Misunderstanding psychoanalysis from the Left." In Robert Samuels, *(Mis)understanding Freud with Lacan, Žižek, and neuroscience.* Springer, 2022: 159–184.
11 Seif, Nancy Gordon. "Otto Rank: On the nature of the hero." *American Imago* 41.4 (1984): 373–384.
12 Blum, Harold P. "Freud and the figure of Moses: The Moses of Freud." *Journal of the American Psychoanalytic Association*39.2 (1991): 513–535.
13 Paul, Robert A. *Moses and civilization: The meaning behind Freud's myth.* Yale University Press, 1996.
14 Holt, Robert R. "On Freud's authoritarianism." *The Psychoanalytic Review* 102.3 (2015): 315–346.
15 Holowchak, Mark. *Freud: From individual psychology to group psychology.* Rowman & Littlefield, 2012.
16 Freeman, Tabitha. "Psychoanalytic concepts of fatherhood: Patriarchal paradoxes and the presence of an absent authority." *Studies in Gender and Sexuality* 9.2 (2008): 113–139.
17 Rice, Emanuel. "Freud, Goethe, and Origen: the duality and slaying of Moses." In L. Bryce Boyer, Ruth M. Boyer, and Stephen M. Sonnenberg (eds.), *The psychoanalytic study of society, volume 18:* Essays in honor of Alan Dundes. Routledge, 2018: 361–380.
18 Rank, Otto. *The myth of the birth of the hero: A psychological exploration of myth.* JHU Press, 2015.
19 Kristeva, Julia. *Strangers to ourselves.* Columbia University Press, 2024.
20 Bernstein, Richard J. *Freud and the Legacy of Moses.* Vol. 4. Cambridge University Press, 1998.

21 Feldman, Arthur A. "Freud's *Moses and Monotheism* and the three stages of Israelitish religion." *The Psychoanalytic Review (1913–1957)* 31 (1944): 361.
22 Schäfer, Peter. "The triumph of pure spirituality: Sigmund Freud's *Moses and Monotheism*." *Jewish Studies Quarterly*9.4 (2002): 381–406.
23 Žižek, Slavoj. "Why should a dialectician learn to count to four?." *Radical Philosophy* 58 (1991): 3–9.
24 Riis, Ole. "Religion re-emerging: the role of religion in legitimating integration and power in modern societies." *International Sociology* 13.2 (1998): 249–272.
25 Tudor, Maya, and Dan Slater. "Nationalism, authoritarianism, and democracy: Historical lessons from South and Southeast Asia." *Perspectives on Politics* 19.3 (2021): 706–722.
26 Freud, Sigmund. *The antithetical meaning of primal words*. Read Books, 2014.
27 Robbins, Michael. "The primary process: Freud's profound yet neglected contribution to the psychology of consciousness." *Psychoanalytic Inquiry* 38.3 (2018): 186–197.
28 Bankirer, Yael Pilowsky. *Psychoanalytic explorations of the masculine and the maternal: Uncovering the image of circumcision in Freud's works*. Routledge, 2024.
29 Donahue, Patricia, and Ellen Quandahl. "Freud and the teaching of interpretation." *College English* 49.6 (1987): 641–649.
30 Samuels, Robert. "Conclusion: Psychoanalysis and the psychology of global enlightenment." In Robert Samuels, *Psychoanalysis and the future of global politics: Overcoming climate change, pandemics, war, and poverty*. Springer, 2023: 93–108.
31 Slavet, Eliza. "Freud's Theory of Jewishness." In Arnold D. Richards (ed.), *The Jewish world of Sigmund Freud: Essays on cultural roots and the problem of religious identity*. McFarland, 2010: 96.
32 Salway, John. "Veritable negroes and circumcised dogs: racial disturbances in Shakespeare." In Lesley Aers and Nigel Wheale (eds.), *Shakespeare in the changing curriculum*. Routledge, 2023: 108–124.
33 Dugan, Holly. "Dispossessed and unaccommodated." In Patricia Akhimie (ed.), *The Oxford handbook of Shakespeare and race*. Oxford University Press, 2024: 339.
34 Lupton, Julia Reinhard. "Ethnos and circumcision in the Pauline tradition: A psychoanalytic exegesis." In Christopher Lane (ed.), *The psychoanalysis of race*. Columbia University Press, 1998: 193–210.
35 Ignatieff, Michael. "Nationalism and toleration." *The Politics of Toleration* 168 (1999): 168.
36 Crossley, James G., and Christian Karner. "Writing history, constructing religion." In James G. Crossley and Christian Karner (eds.). *Writing history, constructing religion*. Routledge, 2018: 3–8.
37 Schwab, Gabriele. "Freud's Moses: Murder, exile, and the question of belonging." In Gilad Sharvit and Karen S. Feldman (eds.), *Freud and monotheism: Moses and the violent origins of religion*. Fordham University Press, 2018: 87–107.
38 Rieff, Philip. *Freud: The mind of the moralist*. University of Chicago Press, 1979.
39 Brockman, Richard. "Freud, Hitler and National Socialism." *The Psychoanalytic Review* 90.5 (2003): 709–722.
40 Johnston, Adrian. "Communism and ambivalence: Freud, Marxism, and aggression." In Jon Mills and Daniel Burston (eds.), *Critical theory and psychoanalysis: From the Frankfurt School to contemporary critique*. Routledge, 2022: 26–65.

41 Miller, Martin A. "Freudian theory under Bolshevik rule: The theoretical controversy during the 1920s." *Slavic Review* 44.4 (1985): 625–646.
42 Foschi, Renato, Marco Innamorati, and Ruggero Taradel. "'A disease of our time': The Catholic Church's condemnation and absolution of psychoanalysis (1924–1975)." *Journal of the History of the Behavioral Sciences* 54.2 (2018): 85–100.
43 Rieff, Philip. *Freud: The mind of the moralist*. University of Chicago Press, 1979.
44 Freud, Sigmund. "Repression." *The Psychoanalytic Review (1913–1957)* 9 (1922): 444.
45 Gaztambide, Daniel José. *A people's history of psychoanalysis: From Freud to liberation psychology*. Rowman & Littlefield, 2019.
46 Adorno, Theodor W., and Max Horkheimer. *Dialectic of enlightenment*. Vol. 15. Verso, 1997.
47 Etchegoyen, Alicia. "Latency—a reappraisal." *The International Journal of Psycho-Analysis* 74.2 (1993): 347.
48 Farley, Helen. "Freud's primal horde: fact or fiction?" *Khthonios: A Journal for the Study of Religion* 1.1 (2003): 32–42.
49 Smith, Richard J. "Darwin, Freud, and the continuing misrepresentation of the primal horde." *Current anthropology*57.6 (2016): 838–843.
50 Bocock, Robert. "The group and the primal horde." In Robert Bocock, *Freud and modern society: An outline and analysis of Freud's sociology*. Springer, 1976: 56–83.
51 Costas, Jana, and Alireza Taheri. "'The return of the primal father' in post-modernity? A Lacanian analysis of authentic leadership." *Organization Studies* 33.9 (2012): 1195–1216.
52 McGrath, William J. "Suggestions and debates: Freud as Hannibal: The politics of the brother band." *Central European History* 7.1 (1974): 31–57.
53 Pulcu, Erdem. "An evolutionary perspective on gradual formation of superego in the primal horde." *Frontiers in Psychology* 5 (2014): 8.
54 Róheim, Géza. "After the death of the primal father." In L. Bryce Boyer and Simon A. Grolnick (eds.), *The psychoanalytic study of society, v. 11: Essays in honor of Werner Muensterberger*. Routledge, 2019: 33–62.
55 Jones, E. "The origin and structure of the super-ego." *The Psychoanalytic Review (1913–1957)* 17 (1930): 55.
56 Sandner, Dieter. "Psychoanalytic considerations of the primal trauma of our culture." In Dieter Sandner, *Society and the unconscious: Cultural psychological insights*. Springer, 2022: 31–40.
57 Smith, Richard J. "Darwin, Freud, and the continuing misrepresentation of the primal horde." *Current Anthropology* 57.6 (2016): 838–843.
58 Bottici, Chiara. "The people and the image of the leader." In Alexander Stagnell, David Payne, and Gustav Strandberg (eds.), *Populism and the people in contemporary critical thought: Politics, philosophy, and aesthetics*. Bloomsbury, 2023: 122.
59 Bottici, Chiara. "Navigating mass psychology: The political myth of Trumpism." In Joshua Branciforte and Ramsey McGlazer (eds.), *Reaction formations: The subject of ethnonationalism*. Oxford University Press, 2021: 58–87.
60 Leeb, Claudia. *Contesting the far right: A psychoanalytic and feminist critical theory approach*. Columbia University Press, 2024.
61 Samuels, Robert. "Understanding the psychopathology of political ideologies." *Psychoanalysis, Culture & Society* 28.2 (2023): 315–323.
62 Birman, Joel. "The political in Freudian discourse." *Research in Psychoanalysis* 21.1 (2016): 85–95.

63 Dean, Jonathan, and Bice Maiguashca. "Gender, power, and left politics: From feminization to 'feministization'." *Politics & Gender* 14.3 (2018): 376–406.
64 Sampson, Anthony. "Freud on the state, violence, and war." *Diacritics* 35.3 (2005): 78–91.
65 Johnson, Pauline. "Feminism and the Enlightenment." *Radical Philosophy* 63 (1993): 3–12.
66 Cavell, Marcia. "Dividing the self." In Gerhard Preyer, Frank Siebelt, and Alexander Ulfig (eds.), *Language, mind and epistemology: On Donald Davidson's philosophy.* Springer, 1994: 299–311.
67 Kristeva, Julia. *Strangers to ourselves.* Columbia University Press, 2024.
68 Homans, Peter. "Disappointment and the ability to mourn: De-idealization as a psychological theme in Freud's life, thought, and social circumstance, 1906–1914." In Paul E. Stepansky (ed.), *Freud, v. 2: Appraisals and reappraisals.* Routledge, 2015: 3–101.
69 Samuels, Robert. "Introduction: Psychoanalysis and future of global progress." In Robert Samuels, *Psychoanalysis and the future of global politics: Overcoming climate change, pandemics, war, and poverty.* Springer, 2023: 1–14.
70 Gresser, Moshe. *Dual allegiance: Freud as a modern Jew.* SUNY Press, 1994.
71 MacLellan, Matthew. "Identity politics, liberalism, and the democratizing power of biopolitics." *Constellations* 28.4 (2021): 555–569.
72 Gilman, Sander L. "Freud, psychoanalysis and antisemitism." In Stephen Frosh and Devorah Baum (eds.), *The Routledge international handbook of psychoanalysis and Jewish studies.* Routledge, 2025: 261–277.
73 Frosh, Stephen. "Psychoanalysis of anti-Semitism II: Splitting and narcissism." In Stephen Frosh, *Hate and the "Jewish science": Anti-Semitism, Nazism and psychoanalysis.* Palgrave Macmillan, 2005: 169–197.
74 Confino, Alon. "Freud, Moses and modern nationhood." In Ruth Ginsburg and Ilana Pardes (eds.), *New perspectives on Freud's "Moses and Monotheism".* De Gruyter, 2006: 165–176.
75 Sachs, Hanns. "'The man Moses' and the man Freud." *The Psychoanalytic Review (1913–1957)* 28 (1941): 156.
76 Santner, Eric L. "Freud's Moses and the ethics of nomotropic desire." *October* (1999): 3–42.
77 Gedo, John E. "Forms of idealization in the analytic transference." *Journal of the American Psychoanalytic Association* 23.3 (1975): 485–505.
78 Schoenfeld, C. G. "God the Father—and Mother: Study and extension of Freud's conception of God as an exalted father." *American Imago* 19.3 (1962): 213–234.
79 Lipman, Matthew, and Salvatore Pizzurro. "Charismatic participation as a sociopathic process." *Psychiatry* 19.1 (1956): 11–30.
80 Gabriel, Yiannis. "Psychoanalytic approaches to leadership." In Alan Bryman, David Collinson, Keith Grint, Brad Jackson, and Mary Uhl-Bien (eds.), *The Sage handbook of leadership.* Sage, 2011: 393–405.
81 Jørstad, Jarl. "Narcissism and leadership: Some differences in male and female leaders." *Nordic Journal of Psychiatry* 49.6 (1995): 409–416.
82 Fonagy, Peter, and Mary Target. "Towards understanding violence: The use of the body and the role of the father." In Rosine Jozef Perelberg (ed.), *Psychoanalytic understanding of violence and suicide.* Routledge, 2005: 45–61.
83 Johnston, Adrian. "The vicious circle of the super-ego: The pathological trap of guilt and the beginning of ethics." *Psychoanalytic Studies* 3.3–4 (2001): 411–424.
84 Batnitzky, Leora. "The image of Judaism: German–Jewish intellectuals and the ban on images." *Jewish Studies Quarterly* 11.3 (2004): 259–281.

85 Assmann, Jan. *The advance in intellectuality: Freud's construction of Judaism*. In Ruth Ginsburg and Ilana Pardes (eds.), *New perspectives on Freud's "Moses and Monotheism"*. De Gruyter, 2006: 7–18.
86 Ragland-Sullivan, Ellie. "The paternal metaphor: a Lacanian theory of language." *Revue Internationale de Philosophie* 46.180 (1992): 49–92.
87 Diamond, Sigmund. "Sigmund Freud, his Jewishness, and scientific method: The seen and the unseen as evidence." *Journal of the History of Ideas* 43.4 (1982): 613–634.
88 Van Herik, Judith. Religion as renunciation and fulfilment: Freud's theories of religion and gender. Dissertation, University of Chicago, 1978.
89 Holt, Robert R. "Freud's impact on modern morality." *Hastings Center Report* (1980): 38–45.
90 Nietzsche, Friedrich. *On the genealogy of morality*. Broadview Press, 2023.
91 Bull, Graham E. "A re-interpretation of a male initiation ritual: Back to Freud via Lacan." *JEP* 3–4 (1996): 1997.
92 Freud, Sigmund. *The future of an illusion*. Broadview Press, 2012.
93 Corveleyn, Jozef. "The psychological explanation of religion as wish-fulfilment. A test-case: The belief in immortality." In Halina Grzymala-Moszczynska and Benjamin Beit-Hallahmi (eds.), *Religion, psychopathology and coping*. Brill, 1996: 57–70.
94 Freud, Sigmund. *Civilization and its discontents*. Broadview Press, 2015.
95 Tambling, Jeremy. "Freud and guilt." In Jeremy Tambling, *Literature and psychoanalysis*. Manchester University Press, 2018: 45–64.
96 Freud, Sigmund. "Mourning and melancholia." In James Strachey (ed.), *The standard edition of the complete psychological works of Sigmund Freud*. Vol. 14. Hogarth Press, 1953–1974: 237–258.
97 Freud, Sigmund. "The economic problem of masochism." *The Psychoanalytic Review* 16 (1929): 209.
98 Inozu, Mujgan, A. Nuray Karanci, and David A. Clark. "Why are religious individuals more obsessional? The role of mental control beliefs and guilt in Muslims and Christians." *Journal of Behavior Therapy and Experimental Psychiatry* 43.3 (2012): 959–966.
99 Horkheimer, Max, and Theodor W. Adorno. *Dialectic of enlightenment*. Stanford University Press, 2002.
100 Kris, Anton O. "The conflicts of ambivalence." *The Psychoanalytic Study of the Child* 39.1 (1984): 213–234.
101 Shalit, Erel. *The hero and his shadow: Psychopolitical aspects of myth and reality in Israel*. Fisher King Press, 2011.
102 Blass, Rachel B. "The role of tradition in concealing and grounding truth: two opposing Freudian legacies on truth and tradition." *American Imago* 63.3 (2006): 331–353.
103 Samuels, Robert. "The future of an illusion and the conservative rejection of globalization." In Robert Samuels, *Psychoanalysis and the future of global politics: Overcoming climate change, pandemics, war, and poverty*. Springer, 2023: 15–31.
104 Samuels, Robert. "The future of an illusion and the conservative rejection of globalization." In Robert Samuels, *Psychoanalysis and the future of global politics: Overcoming climate change, pandemics, war, and poverty*. Springer, 2023: 15–31.
105 Agley, Jon. "Assessing changes in US public trust in science amid the COVID-19 pandemic." *Public Health* 183 (2020): 122–125.
106 Peng, Yilang. "Give me liberty or give me COVID-19: How social dominance orientation, right-wing authoritarianism, and libertarianism explain Americans' reactions to COVID-19." *Risk Analysis* 42.12 (2022): 2691–2703.

107 Van Prooijen, Jan-Willem, and André PM Krouwel. "Psychological features of extreme political ideologies." *Current Directions in Psychological Science* 28.2 (2019): 159–163.
108 Baker, Susan D., et al. "The role of trust and communication in fostering followers' self perceptions as leaders." *Journal of Managerial Issues* 28.3–4 (2016): 210–230.
109 Paul, Robert A. *Moses and civilization: The meaning behind Freud's myth*. Yale University Press, 1996.
110 Grossman, William I. "Hierarchies, boundaries, and representation in a Freudian model of mental organization." *Journal of the American Psychoanalytic Association* 40.1 (1992): 27–62.
111 Young, Allan. "Remembering the evolutionary Freud." *Science in Context* 19.1 (2006): 175–189.
112 Freud, Sigmund. *The ego and the id*. Simon and Schuster, 2019. Hereafter cited as "*EI*" in this chapter.
113 Lapsley, Daniel K., and Paul C. Stey. "Id, ego, and superego." In V. S. Ramachandran (ed.), *Encyclopedia of Human Behavior*, 2nd edition. Elsevier, 2011: 1–9.
114 Freud, Sigmund. "Formulations on the two principles of mental functioning." In Riccardo Steiner (ed.), *Unconscious phantasy*. Routledge, 2018: 67–76.
115 Samuels, Robert. "Science and the reality principle." In Robert Samuels, *Freud for the twenty-first century: The science of everyday life*. Springer, 2019: 5–16.
116 Singer, Jerome L. "Delayed gratification and ego development: implications for clinical and experimental research." *Journal of Consulting Psychology* 19.4 (1955): 259.
117 Loewald, Hans W. "Ego and reality." *The International Journal of Psycho-Analysis* 32 (1951): 10.
118 Schur, Max. "The ego and the id in anxiety." *The Psychoanalytic Study of the Child* 13.1 (1958): 190–220.
119 Doidge, Norman. "Classics revisited: Freud's 'The ego and the id' and 'Inhibitions, Symptoms and Anxiety'." *Journal of the American Psychoanalytic Association* 50.1 (2002): 281–294.
120 Helminen, Vilja, Marko Elovainio, and Markus Jokela. "Clinical symptoms of anxiety disorders as predictors of political attitudes: A prospective cohort study." *International Journal of Psychology* 57.2 (2022): 181–189.
121 Leahy, Michael P. T. "Neutrality." *Metaphilosophy* 5.3 (1974): 181–186.
122 Freud, Anna. "The mutual influences in the development of ego and id: Introduction to the discussion." *The Psychoanalytic Study of the Child* 7.1 (1952): 42–50.
123 Clark, L, Pierce. "A psychological study of sycophancy." *The Psychoanalytic Review (1913–1957)* 21 (1934): 15.
124 Pardos-Prado, Sergi. "How can mainstream parties prevent niche party success? Center-right parties and the immigration issue." *The Journal of Politics* 77.2 (2015): 352–367.
125 Samuels, Robert. "Cancel culture, free speech, and the center-Right." In Robert Samuels, *Culture wars, universities, and the political unconscious*. Springer, 2024: 59–76.
126 Sperber, Joshua. "The political economy of the podcast and the rise of the left entrepreneur." *Ephemera* 21.4 (2021): 249–264.
127 Haidt, Jonathan. "Why concepts creep to the left." *Psychological Inquiry* 27.1 (2016): 40–45.
128 Samuels, Robert, and Robert Samuels. "Catharsis: The politics of enjoyment." In Robert Samuels, *Žižek and the rhetorical unconscious: Global politics, philosophy, and subjectivity*. Springer, 2020: 7–31.

129 Whynacht, Ardath J. "Citizens of nowhere": Diffractive engagements with borderline personality disorder. Dissertation, Concordia University, 2017.
130 Sirkin, Mark, and Michael Fleming. "Freud's 'project' and its relationship to psychoanalytic theory." *Journal of the History of the Behavioral Sciences* 18.3 (1982): 230–241.
131 Meissner, William W. "Notes on identification: I. Origins in Freud." *The Psychoanalytic Quarterly* 39.4 (1970): 563–589.
132 Klein, Melanie. "Early stages of the Oedipus conflict." In Russell Grigg, Dominique Hecq, and Craig Smith (eds.), *Female sexuality: The Early Psychoanalytic Controversies*. Routledge, 2018: 146–158.
133 Bronfenbrenner, Urie. "Freudian theories of identification and their derivatives." *Child Development* 31.1 (1960): 15–40.
134 Britzman, Deborah P. "A Note to 'Identification with the aggressor'." *Counterpoints* 300 (2006): 41–59.
135 Borch-Jacobsen, Mikkel, and Douglas Brick. "The Oedipus problem in Freud and Lacan." *Critical Inquiry* 20.2 (1994): 267–282.
136 Homayounpour, Gohar. "*The Ego and the Id* and … the superego." In Fred Busch and Natacha Delgado (eds.), *The ego and the Id: 100 Years Later*. Routledge, 2023: 25–31.
137 Morrison, Andrew P. "Shame, ideal self, and narcissism." *Contemporary Psychoanalysis* 19.2 (1983): 295–318.
138 Hanly, Charles. "Ego ideal and ideal ego." *The International Journal of Psycho-Analysis* 65 (1984): 253.
139 Cook, Deborah. "Foucault, Freud, and the repressive hypothesis." *Journal of the British Society for Phenomenology* 45.2 (2014): 148–161.
140 Chodorow, Nancy J. *Femininities, masculinities, sexualities: Freud and beyond*. University Press of Kentucky, 2014.
141 Groot, Jeanne Lampl-De. "Ego ideal and superego." *The Psychoanalytic Study of the Child* 17.1 (1962): 94–106.
142 Daley, James W. "Freud: The ethics of ambivalence." *The Intercollegiate Review* 13.1 (1977): 45.
143 Freud, Sigmund. *Group psychology and the analysis of the ego*. Hogarth Press, 1949.
144 Kitcher, Patricia. "Kant's conscience and Freud's super-ego." In Stefanie Grüne and Colin Marshall (eds.), *Kant's lasting legacy: Essays in Honor of Béatrice Longuenesse*. Routledge, 2025: 207–223.
145 Van Herik, Judith. Religion as renunciation and fulfilment: Freud's theories of religion and gender. Dissertation, University of Chicago, 1978.
146 Spruiell, Vann. "Freud's concepts of idealization." *Journal of the American Psychoanalytic Association* 27.4 (1979): 777–791.
147 Bergmann, Martin S. "Moses and the evolution of Freud's Jewish identity." In Mortimer Ostow (ed.), *Judaism and psychoanalysis*. Routledge, 2018: 111–142.
148 Oppenheim, Michael. "Loving the neighbor: Some reflections on narcissism." *Modern Judaism* 27.1 (2007): 47–71.
149 Figlio, Karl. "The dread of sameness: Social hatred and Freud's 'narcissism of minor differences'." By Lene Auestad (ed.), *Psychoanalysis and politics: Exclusion and the politics of representation*. Routledge, 2012: 29–46.
150 Etchegoyen, Alicia. "Psychoanalytic ideas about fathers." In Alicia Etchegoyen and Judith Trowell (eds.), *The importance of fathers: A Psychoanalytic Re-evaluation*. Routledge, 2005: 18–37.
151 Sandler, Joseph, Alex Holder, and Dale Meers. "The ego ideal and the ideal self." *The Psychoanalytic Study of the Child* 18.1 (1963): 139–158.

152 Moncayo, Raul Leon. The moral unconscious and the dimension of the other: An inquiry into Freud's intrapsychic theory of repression. Dissertation, The Wright Institute, 1985.
153 Samuels, Robert. "(Liberal) Narcissism." In Yannis Stavrakakis (ed.), *Routledge handbook of psychoanalytic political theory*. Routledge, 2019: 151–161.
154 Wallace, Edwin R. "Freud as ethicist." In Paul E. Stepansky (ed.), *Freud, v. 1: Appraisals and reappraisals*. Routledge, 2015: 83–141.
155 Tambling, Jeremy. "Freud and guilt." In Jeremy Tambling, *Literature and psychoanalysis*. Manchester University Press, 2018: 45–64.
156 Gellis, André, and Maria Isabel Lima Hamud. "Sense of guilt in Freudian work: Universal and unconscious." *Psicologia USP* 22 (2011): 635–654.
157 Sillman, Leonard R. "The analysis of guilt and narcissism." *The Journal of Nervous and Mental Disease* 133.4 (1961): 293–302.
158 Freud, Sigmund. "Mourning and melancholia." *The Psychoanalytic Review* 11 (1924): 77.
159 Kanaan, Richard A. "Hysteria and the varieties of deception." *AJOB Neuroscience* 1.1 (2010): 55–64.
160 Samuels, Robert, and Robert Samuels. "Pathos, hysteria, and the Left." In Robert Samuels, *Žižek and the rhetorical unconscious: Global politics, philosophy, and subjectivity*. Springer, 2020: 33–47.
161 Colbach, Edward M. "Hysteria again and again and again." *International Journal of Offender Therapy and Comparative Criminology* 31.1 (1987): 41–48.
162 Decker, Hannah S. "Freud and Dora: Constraints on medical progress." *Journal of Social History* 14.3 (1981): 445–464.
163 Jennings, Jerry L. "Freud's case of Dora: Wellspring of discovery and discourse." *Open Journal of Social Sciences* 10.1 (2022): 290–314.
164 Benvenuto, Sergio. "Freud and masochism." *European Journal of Psychoanalysis* 16 (2003).
165 Chabert, Catherine. "Plural feminine: Hysteria, masochism or melancholia?." *The International Journal of Psychoanalysis* 100.3 (2019): 584–592.
166 Feyerabend, Paul K. "On the critique of scientific reason." *Essays in memory of Imre Lakatos*. Springer, 1976: 109–143.

Conclusion

Throughout this book, one goal has been to increase our understanding of the diverse ideologies shaping the world today. In relating particular ideologies to specific psychopathologies and mental agencies, I have used Freud's theories to base each belief system on the extreme form of a basic human relational desire.[1] Thus, libertarian ideology is derived from the call to be free from social regulation and mental tension, while authoritarian ideology relies on the desire for salvation. Since one wants to be saved by an idealized object, one suspends one's own reality-testing ego. In this structure, we find the dominance of the object through a process of transference, but in the case of libertarian ideology, it is the drives in the id that dominate.[2] Moreover, in the case of the ideology of traditionalism, social morality and order is imposed with the internalization of the super-ego.[3] Through the combination of projection, introjection, and prediction, we find paranoid knowledge and conspiracy theories.[4]

While Freud posits that humans are driven by the pleasure principle, which calls for the release of all mental tension, conservatives experience this tension as anxiety when they are unable to predict what will happen next.[5] Faced with an uncertain future, conservatives experience panic caused by the triggering of an evolutionary fight-or-flight mechanism.[6] To counteract this anxiety, they make a call for protection, which often results in blaming some out-group for destabilizing the social order.[7] It is vital to stress here that most examinations of contemporary politics do not differentiate between conservative, authoritarian, and traditionalist ideologies. They also tend to conflate the libertarian Right with other anti-Left ideologies.[8]

In the case of the Left, we discover how the expression of suffering is often used to form an identity and to make a call for accommodation. In fact, many minority-based social movements are centered on presenting the unfair treatment of disempowered groups.[9] While the Left, then, seeks accommodation, what we find in the center-Left is a desire to be admired for one's good intentions.[10] As a way to verify the ideal ego, center-Left narcissists signal their virtue as they repress their underlying anti-social desires, guilt, and shame.[11] Meanwhile, in the case of the center-Right, we find people who

DOI: 10.4324/9781003773948-9

want to be seen as being liberal and rational, when in fact, they are pursuing and rationalizing their privilege.[12]

As a key aspect of global progress, liberalism brings together the desire for truth and the call for equality.[13] Although some may say that this ideology is really an anti-ideology, we must affirm that the ideals of neutrality and universality do not exist in nature, and so they are necessary but impossible human goals that we strive to attain.[14] In fact, when I first started writing this book, my aim was to show why we need to replace the seven other ideologies mentioned above with liberal ideology in order to resolve global problems and develop a sense of global identity and consciousness. However, I now believe that this project is doomed because one cannot simply move beyond the underlying desires shaping the other ideologies. Thus, it is necessary to find a way to moderate and balance the different relational desires driving distinct belief systems. In other words, we have to integrate the desires for freedom, order, salvation, admiration, protection, accommodation, innocence, and truth together.

One reason why this integration is necessary is that we have seen how each ideology relates to the dominance of a particular mental agency, and so we cannot simply ignore these fundamental human thought processes. However, what we can do is to cater to the non-extreme form of these different desires and agencies.[15] Thus, instead of simply promoting the freedom of the isolated individual, we must show a respect for individual rights as we balance these by the need for universal laws.[16] Likewise, we have to recognize the desires for protection and social order, but we have to do this without relying on conspiracy theories or the stigmatization of out-groups.[17] We also have to trust others yet also verify what they are saying.[18] Furthermore, we have to find ways of helping disadvantaged people without feeding a victim identity, and it is also necessary to admire the good intentions of people, while still realizing that we have to judge them by what they do and not what they say.

As we see with the issue of climate change, we know what should be done, and we have the rational science to prove it, yet many people either ignore the issue or don't know how to fix it.[19] Of course, one of the reasons why a global solution is not being promoted is that we continue to use national politics and policies to deal with issues that are global. Since we lack a strong form of global governance and enforcement, it is impossible to resolve issues like climate change, pandemics, AI, genetic modification, immigration, taxation, and finance.[20] Moreover, the different ideologies mentioned in this book all act to undermine the need for some form of global democracy because they do not take an integrated approach to the human mind and social organization.[21] Since each ideology represents an extreme form of a particular desire and agency, it is necessary to tie the creation of globalism to the moderation and balancing of these diverse needs.

While this book has not spent a great deal of time discussing what I mean by globalism, the main idea is that we need a type of thinking and social organization that begins with an international perspective.[22] As a form of consciousness, the idea is that we value the lives of everyone in the world on an equal basis, but we also value the different competing desires that structure our humanity. By affirming that we are all part of an integrated system, and what we do affects everyone else, we can begin to affirm a global mode of consciousness.[23]

Notes

1 Samuels, Robert. *The psychopathology of political ideologies.* Routledge, 2021.
2 Iyer, Ravi, et al. "Understanding libertarian morality: The psychological roots of an individualist ideology." *PLoS One* 7.8 (2010): e42366.
3 Tsekeris, Charalambos. "Chaos and unpredictability in social thought: General considerations and perspectives." *Sociologija* 2 (2010): 34–47.
4 Mills, Jon. "Lacan on paranoiac knowledge." In Jon Mills and David L. Downing (eds.), *Lacan on psychosis.* Routledge, 2018: 10–46.
5 Castano, Emanuele, et al. "Ideology, fear of death, and death anxiety." *Political Psychology* 32.4 (2011): 601–621.
6 Mendez, Mario F. "A neurology of the conservative-liberal dimension of political ideology." *The Journal of Neuropsychiatry and Clinical Neurosciences* 29.2 (2017): 86–94.
7 Gentry, Caron E. "Anxiety and the creation of the scapegoated other." *Critical Studies on Security* 3.2 (2015): 133–146.
8 Klein, Ezra. *Why we're polarized.* Simon and Schuster, 2020.
9 Freeman, Samuel. "Liberalism and the accommodation of group claims." In Paul Kelly (ed.), *Multiculturalism reconsidered.* Wiley, 2002: 18–30.
10 Liu, Catherine. *Virtue hoarders: The case against the professional managerial class.* U of Minnesota Press, 2021.
11 Samuels, Robert. "Beyond Hillary Clinton: obsessional narcissism and the failure of the liberal class." In Robert Samuels, *Psychoanalyzing the Left and Right after Donald Trump: Conservatism, liberalism, and neoliberal populisms.* Springer, 2016: 31–59.
12 Samuels, Robert. "Cancel culture, free speech, and the center-Right." In Robert Samuels, *Culture wars, universities, and the political unconscious.* Springer, 2024: 59–76.
13 Pagden, Anthony. *The Enlightenment: and why it still matters.* Oxford University Press, 2013.
14 Samuels, Robert. "The Left's Critique of Psychoanalysis and Globalization." In Robert Samuels, *Psychoanalysis and the future of global politics: Overcoming climate change, pandemics, war, and poverty.* Springer, 2023: 33–49.
15 Van Prooijen, Jan-Willem, and André PM Krouwel. "Psychological features of extreme political ideologies." *Current Directions in Psychological Science* 28.2 (2019): 159–163.
16 Foldvary, Fred E. *The soul of liberty: The universal ethic of freedom and human rights.* Gutenberg Press, 1980.
17 Rawal, Nabin. "Social inclusion and exclusion: A review." *Dhaulagiri Journal of Sociology and Anthropology* 2 (2008): 161–180.
18 Gundlach, Gregory T., and Joseph P. Cannon. "'Trust but verify'? The performance implications of verification strategies in trusting relationships." *Journal of the Academy of Marketing Science* 38 (2010): 399–417.

19 Dunlap, Riley E., and Aaron M. McCright. "Climate change denial: Sources, actors and strategies." In Steven R. Brechin and Seungyun Lee (eds.), *Routledge handbook of climate change and society.* Routledge, 2010: 240–259.
20 Halliday, Fred. "Global governance: prospects and problems." *Citizenship studies* 4.1 (2000): 19–33.
21 Weiss, Thomas G. *Global governance: Why? what? whither?* John Wiley & Sons, 2016.
22 Robertson, Roland. "Global connectivity and global consciousness." *American Behavioral Scientist* 55.10 (2011): 1336–1345.
23 Mansilla, Veronica Boix, and Howard Gardner. "From teaching globalization to nurturing global consciousness." In Marcelo M. Suárez-Orozco (ed.), *Learning in the global era: International perspectives on globalization and education.* University of California Press, 2007: 47–66.

Index

For Product Safety Concerns and Information please contact our EU
representative GPSR@taylorandfrancis.com
Taylor & Francis Verlag GmbH, Kaufingerstraße 24, 80331 München, Germany

www.ingramcontent.com/pod-product-compliance
Ingram Content Group UK Ltd.
Pitfield, Milton Keynes, MK11 3LW, UK
UKHW020002200926
475702UK00015B/2429

* 9 7 8 1 0 4 1 3 0 3 2 1 3 *